THE ULTIMATE RAPE

What Every Woman Should Know About Hysterectomies and Ovarian Removal

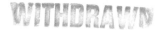
Elizabeth L. Plourde, M.T., M.A.

PUBLISHER'S NOTE:

Where first names are used to identify an individual in the text of this book, these names are pseudonyms only.

AN IMPORTANT CAUTION TO OUR READERS:

This book is not a medical manual and cannot take the place of personalized medical advice and treatment from a qualified physician. The reader should regularly consult a physician in matters relating to his or her health, particularly with respect to any symptoms that may require diagnosis or treatment. Although certain medical procedures and medical professionals are mentioned in this book, no endorsement, warranty or guarantee by the author is intended. Every attempt has been made to ensure that the information contained in this book is current, however, due to the fact that research is ongoing, some of the material may be invalidated by new findings. The author and publisher cannot guarantee that the information and advice in this book are safe and proper for every reader. For that reason, this book is sold without warranties or guarantees of any kind, expressed or implied, and the author and publisher disclaim any liability, loss or damage caused by the contents. If you do not wish to be bound by these cautions and conditions, you may return your copy to the publisher for a full refund.

Library of Congress Catalog-in Publication Data

Plourde, Elizabeth L.
The Ultimate Rape: What Every Woman Should Know about Hysterectomies and Ovarian Removal/Elizabeth L. Plourde
Includes bibliographic references & index

ISBN 0-9661735-0-3   LCCN 97-92836

Cover illustration: James Kelley
Editing: Virginia Schmidt

Published in the United States by
New Voice Publications
P.O. Box 14133
Irvine, CA 92623-4133

This book is dedicated to:

My daughter, Wendy Protzman, who had to become her own mother for years; not only as a result of my surgery, but also throughout the time I spent researching and writing this book.

My mother, Virginia Schmidt, whose steadfast enthusiastic support, tireless editing, and gifted way with words were invaluable contributions to this work.

My husband, Marcus, whose understanding, support, and 100% commitment to what turned out to be a second edition, even before the first printing, helped speed the process of bringing this important message to all women.

Acknowledgments

This book has been such a long journey, it is difficult to include all the people who have helped along the way. I could not have finished this project without the overwhelming support I received from my entire family and many friends. I am truly grateful and feel incredibly blessed by their unending encouragement, especially when this book has taken 100% of my time for so many years.

I extend my deepest gratitude to all the women throughout the years who, by sharing their stories, opened the doors to the topics I researched and covered in this book. Their experiences helped add to my awareness, not only of the complexity and individuality of our bodies, but also to the wide range of reactions that follow these surgeries.

Many heartfelt thanks go to my editors; Virginia Schmidt, Marcus Plourde, and Anita Porter, who so gladly and freely gave of their time to help produce an easily read and understood finished product.

I extend special acknowledgment and thanks to my nephew, James Kelley. His creative expertise brought my vision of the dust jacket to life.

I am grateful to Dr. William Fullerton, Dr. Robert Green, and Dr. James Wooley for their helpful advice at various stages of the manuscript.

The librarians at UCLA and University of California, Irvine also deserve special mention, especially April Love. Her friendly direction not only sped up the thousands of hours spent in the library, but also helped make the time much more enjoyable.

Most of all, my deepest thanks go to my husband, Marcus, who bore the pain of the book's birthing process right along with me. No words can truly express the appreciation I feel for the understanding and belief in this project he extended throughout the entire process.

I especially thank God for the opportunity and resources that have been provided to bring this book to print.

Elizabeth Plourde
September 1998

TABLE OF CONTENTS

All Truth Passes Through 3 Stages

- First: It is ridiculous

- Second: It is violently opposed

- Third: It is accepted as being self-evident

—Schopenhauer

Prologue

While listening to a talk radio program, I heard a woman caller who sounded as depressed and "shook to her core" as I was after my hysterectomy. The description she relayed of what her life had been like since her surgery sounded exactly like mine. I heard her pain and her agony. The despair in her voice gave me, not only the impetus to begin, but also the energy to keep writing this book. No one should have to endure what this woman and I have gone through. The truth about the complications that can arise from hysterectomies needs to be told. The experience of millions is vastly different from what many doctors convey when recommending this surgery. Both hysterectomized and non-hysterectomized women, alike, deserve the opportunity to learn how their bodies can be affected by the removal of their childbearing organs.

Introduction

I wrote the book I wish had been available before I said "yes" to this "life-changing" operation. The books I read prior to surgery presented the potential consequences in such a dry, insignificant, and scientific manner, I felt there was no need for concern. I know now that if the information contained in this book had been accessible to me, I would have explored other options.

As a result of my surgery, I suffered both physical and emotional devastation for almost two years before finding a doctor who understood that my symptoms were caused by the loss of hormones and chemicals produced by the ovaries and uterus. Throughout those difficult years, every doctor I saw told me all my problems must be in my head, and that I should see a psychiatrist. Fortunately, when I finally found a doctor who recognized my hormone-deficient state, she immediately placed me on a hormone replacement program that gradually returned me to my original self.

When I bounced back to life, I wanted to know more about what had happened to me. What did the hormone loss really mean to my body, and how could I protect myself against future problems? Part of my professional career involved researching medical journals to assist busy doctors in quickly accessing the latest research, so I decided to use this knowledge and expertise to find help for my surgically-altered state.

As I started reading the research and medical journals

published world-wide, the information dumfounded me. I was astonished to find out how much the medical community knows, but does not convey to women about their own bodies. I was equally amazed to discover that every symptom I experienced had been linked to hysterectomies since the 1930s, a half a century before my 1985 surgery.

Article after article led me to many new forks in the road— forks that revealed there are a multitude of possible consequences which can arise out of this surgery, some immediately apparent, and some which take years to silently develop. When my literature search proved altered biochemistry creates these devastating effects, and that they potentially place every surgically compromised woman's health in jeopardy, I knew I had to bring this information to the awareness of all women, everywhere.

It has been a lack of understanding about our bodies' incredible complexity that has allowed the philosophy:

> *A woman's reproductive organs are only good for one thing—childbearing—and after a woman has had all the children she wants, these precious organs are expendable.*

This idea became rooted during a time when the available technology could not identify the many functions performed by the uterus and ovaries, and no studies were conducted to determine the validity of such a belief. Yet, throughout the 20th century, doctors have been trained to view a hysterectomy as: *The best thing that could ever happen to a woman.*

These misconceptions have resulted in the practice of hysterectomies becoming a world-wide phenomenon, with the United States, Canada, and Australia performing them at rates higher than anywhere else in the world.[1] This high rate has led to hysterectomies becoming the second most frequently performed major surgical operation in America. As a result, over 500,000 women elect for surgical removal of their uterus as a cure for many female problems every year. In addition, the fear of developing cancer has led to nearly 300,000 of these women sacrificing their ovaries at the same time.[2]

Today, however, advanced research techniques irrefutably prove the deterioration that occurs within women's bodies when they lose the natural protection of their hormones. They also demonstrate how the ovaries produce essential chemicals throughout a woman's life, even past menopause, and clearly reveal why hysterectomized women become higher risk, long-term health care patients.

This book is the culmination of 12 years of research. Throughout this time, as I critically evaluated each journal article, something was lacking in so many of the studies, I was compelled to return to the libraries to do even more extensive research. What I found was that a large percentage of the studies which have been conducted so far have not been designed, either to answer the questions women have, or to provide the information they need regarding the full impact of organ removal on their bodies. As a result, after analyzing well over 30,000 medical and research articles, they were ultimately distilled down to the 856 citations listed.

Presented in an easy-to-understand format, this book represents the most current material available today. Its chapters contain vital information women need when confronted with the question of whether to have a hysterectomy, or their ovaries prophylactically removed. Only after being fully informed about the many short and long-term consequences can they make the decision as to whether utilizing a hysterectomy to alleviate their current symptoms is worth the risks involved. Women have a right to know these facts beforehand—because their surgery cannot be reversed, their organs cannot be restored, nor can their own personal hormone factories be duplicated, or replaced, EVER.

One doctor stated that women can act on their own behalf by asking the right questions. In reality, without an awareness and understanding of the numerous and far-reaching new problems that can result from these surgeries, it is impossible for women to know the "right" questions to ask. Therefore, this book is dedicated to providing women with the "right" questions to ask, either before or after surgery: before, so they will explore other options more intensively; or after, enabling women to take steps to protect their bodies, so they will not be surprised by heart attacks or osteoporotic broken bones, way too early in life.

We can no longer afford to ignore the harmful effects and extensive costs, which result from stripping women of their health-maintaining reproductive organs. In addition to empowering women to become educated consumers about their own bodies, this book is a wake-up call, exposing the true burden that this "standard medical practice" places on women's bodies; ultimately affecting their lives, those of their families, our health care systems, and society as a whole. It is also written with the hope that other women will never have to feel as I still do—wishing I had never had the surgery.

As part of your reading, please include a review of the reference notes at the end of the book. The article titles, alone, tell the story of how detrimental hysterectomies are for the human body.

THE ULTIMATE RAPE

**What Every Woman Should Know About
Hysterectomies and Ovarian Removal**

1

Waking Up:
Hysterectomy Discoveries

"Elizabeth, . . . Elizabeth, . . . you have to wake up!" These faint words appeared to be coming from far away, through a dense cloud. As I attempted to move, a stabbing pain in my abdomen stopped me short. Bleary-eyed, I tried to focus on the person who was shaking my shoulder and calling my name. Where was I? Who was talking? Gradually becoming conscious, I realized I was in a hospital room, and a nurse was telling me to swallow the pill she held next to my lips. Still so groggy from the anesthetic I had received for abdominal surgery, I did not understand why I needed a pill. Weakly, I asked, "What is it for?"

She answered, "It is an estrogen pill. The doctor removed your ovaries and left orders to give you estrogen right away, to prevent hot flushes."

Even through my thick fog, her answer baffled me. I felt confused. I had signed a release for a hysterectomy, but I understood the rest was supposed to be exploratory only. Why did the doctor take my ovaries? How could they have been causing the pain I had been experiencing? Too weak to do anything else, I swallowed the pill and drifted back under the spell of the anesthetic.

That evening, when the doctor checked in on me, I asked, "Why did you remove my ovaries?"

He replied, "You not only had varicose veins in your

uterus, you also had varicose veins wrapped around one ovary. So, since you are over 40, and don't need your ovaries anymore, I decided to take them out at the same time, to save you from ovarian cancer."

I was incredulous—too stunned to respond. I thought to myself, What do you mean I don't need them any more, when the estrogen they produce is so critical that you have the nurse rouse me from anesthesia to ensure I do not feel their loss! I was too sore, weak, and confused to do more than meekly accept what had been done. After all, how could I challenge a doctor? He must have known what he was doing.

The next day when I discovered there were stitches in my vaginal opening, I asked the doctor why they were there. He replied that he had taken advantage of the fact that I was already under anesthesia, so why not, at the same time, cut the length of my vagina and resew it tighter. If I was amazed at both my ovaries being gone, this new revelation made me even more incredulous.

I exclaimed, "You never mentioned this prior to surgery!"

The doctor responded, "This is the normal thing to do. I just operated on a ninety-year-old woman who had a vaginal prolapse due to her stretched vagina. You wouldn't want that in the future, would you?"

So, he decided to take it upon himself to save me from such an experience. How could he have performed these procedures without my knowledge and consent? Prior to surgery we had only agreed upon a hysterectomy. Neither the possibility of the removal of my ovaries, nor the cutting of my vagina were discussed. Needing to understand how these things had happened, I thought back over the events leading to this operation.

The cramps I experienced during each period were manageable, but the excruciating pain that came and went throughout the month doubled me over at times. When it happened while I was driving, I would have to pull over to the side of the road until it passed.

In addition, during my period, bath towels were the only thing thick enough to absorb the heavy flow. When the excessive bleeding started, the doctor tested my estrogen levels. After informing me that, at the age of 40 I was entering menopause, he offered to give me supplemental estrogen if I wanted it. Hoping this was an easy answer, I agreed to try it. At the same time, he ordered an ultrasound of my ovaries, the results of which indicated they were normal.

As months went by, there was no change in the bleeding or the pain. When I saw the doctor again, his response was, "The only answer left is a hysterectomy. Consider it."

It was hard to face the thought of another surgery. I knew from having my gallbladder removed seven years earlier, that no matter what doctors say, recovery time is difficult. As a single mother trying to raise a seven year old daughter, I could not afford the time off work, nor risk losing my job.

When I did not opt for surgery, we kept trying to correct these problems with estrogen. After three more years of this therapy, I was still bleeding profusely, as well as doubling over in pain. Needing to find relief somehow, I made another doctor's appointment. The blood work he had ordered still indicated abnormally low estrogen levels, making the doctor reiterate that I was in early menopause. He stated again that a hysterectomy would solve my bleeding, and in addition he could explore to see what was causing my pain.

Before submitting to another surgery, I consulted with a woman gynecologist for a second opinion, as well as for any possible alternatives.

She concurred that a hysterectomy was my "only" avenue of relief, and emphasized how much better life would be afterward. Feeling I had no other options and nowhere else to turn, I finally consented to the operation.

Now, while laying in my hospital bed, even though the extent of the surgery left me in a state of shock, I knew I had to face the reality that the procedures were irreversible. My only choice left was to accept what had been done. After all, my reproductive organs could not be put back into my body. They were gone for good. As a result, I rationalized that the doctor's solution must have been the right one, and what had happened was for the best.

On the way home from the hospital, I told myself that all I have to do now is recover, and begin looking forward to a pain-free life, one that would be free of the inconvenience of trying to work during my menstrual period.

Over the next few months, however, life was entirely different from what I had expected. True, the hysterectomy eliminated the excessive bleeding every month, but I was experiencing many changes that my doctors never discussed with me prior to surgery. First, there was no difference in the amount of pain, and the intensity still doubled me over at times. For several weeks, I passed it off, assuming it was from the healing of the scar tissue. Although, as the months passed, this explanation could no longer justify the crippling, recurring pain. Second, I was becoming increasingly depressed, unlike anything I had ever felt before in my life. The third, very apparent change, was that I had lost all interest in sex. Feeling asexual, I felt sex had become a waste of time.

Concerned about what was happening to me, I dragged myself to the doctor's office. Describing what life had been like over the last few months, I related to the doctor, "My pain has not changed, I feel overwhelmed by a growing depression, and sexually I cannot respond at all. I'm making excuses to avoid sex, rather than to submit to something that I can no longer feel."

He responded, "First, you cannot be in pain, I removed everything. Second, the depression could be the result of having difficulty adjusting to the loss of your organs. Maybe you should see a psychiatrist." He then asked me how my sex life had been before the surgery.

My answer was, "Fabulous!"

"Why didn't you tell me this prior to surgery?" he asked.

Amazed, I replied, "Why should I have brought up something that was working well? I had no reason to discuss it."

His incomprehensible reply was, "I guess I should have asked you about it before we operated." Too stunned to speak, I thought, is he implying that this is the way I will be for the rest of my life? Asexual?

He continued, "Well, you are taking estrogen, maybe you also need testosterone. We believe the ovaries make about 13 different chemicals, although not all of them have been identified. We do know one is testosterone, which is what accounts for men's stronger sex drive." Thinking it would help, the doctor gave me a testosterone shot before I left his office.

At this point, in an attempt to understand what was happening to me, I pulled out my college textbooks to read about testosterone. Since ovaries are the counterpart to men's testicles, they do produce testosterone, although in smaller amounts. The books confirmed that testosterone is responsible for everyone's sexual drive, male or female. By now, my lack of sexual response was so pronounced, I realized that even though women produce smaller amounts, what they do produce is essential for them.

A few days after the testosterone shot I developed a rash all over my body. When I reported this to the doctor, his only answer was, "It is obvious you cannot take testosterone. I have no other options available for you." With my new understanding of the important roll that testosterone plays in our bodies, I became discouraged that I would never be able to artificially replace this critical hormone.

As the weeks dragged on, my depression grew deeper by the day. I became lethargic and began not wanting to leave the house. I even started to feel suicidal. Terrified of these thoughts, I called my doctor begging for help. Again, he reiterated that maybe what I really needed was to see a psychiatrist. "No," I insisted, "it is not in my head. I am feeling an imbalance in my body; an imbalance over which I seem to have no control." He had no answer for me and defended his removal of my ovaries as being a standard procedure for all women over 40. As a last resort, he said he would contact the experts at the local university medical center, asking them about his decision to take my ovaries, and to obtain information about any possible help for me. We set up an appointment to discuss his findings.

When we met, he reported, "The experts substantiated what I learned in medical school. They concurred that if you open up a women over 40, for her own safety, and to insure that she will not develop ovarian cancer in the future, it is best to take her ovaries." He explained that this was "standard medical practice" and asked, "Would you want to risk developing ovarian cancer in the future?" Amplifying the fear, he added, "By the time women are diagnosed with ovarian cancer, it is usually too late."

As I left his office, I pondered over what "standard medical practice" meant. In this case, it meant removing perfectly healthy, normal organs, only out of fear that they might become diseased at some time in the "future", thereby putting the patient's "present" quality of life "at risk." This did not make sense to me. I found myself wishing I could go back and undo the surgery.

By now, more confused than ever, it became obvious to me that I needed to know more about hysterectomies and their effects on the body. I went to the university medical center library and started reading all I could about hysterectomies, oophorectomies (removal of the ovaries), and ovarian cancer. I was grateful for the education that I had acquired to become licensed as a Medical Technologist, and for the professional training in medical research I received while selling cutting-edge technology to doctors. These experiences provided the necessary background to understand the technical medical journals.

Everything I read confirmed what I was experiencing. I found studies proving that approximately 30% of women develop depression following a hysterectomy. Additionally, articles published well before my surgery warned about the loss of sexual response following hysterectomies. Again, I asked myself, why hadn't my doctor discussed these potential outcomes with me? Obviously, he had known about the possible loss of sex drive, or he wouldn't have said that he "should" have asked about my sex life before the operation.

I made another appointment with the doctor to discuss my findings. After reviewing the material, he agreed with their conclusions, but confessed that he did not know how to help me. Since he had limited formal training in the complex inter-relationship of the hormones in the body, his only recourse was to refer me to an endocrinologist (a hormone specialist).

With renewed hope, I met with the endocrinologist. We discussed my depression and loss of sexual response. His answer for the depression was to prescribe a different brand of estrogen, combined with progesterone and thyroid hormones. As far as addressing my lack of sexual response, this new specialist's blithe answer was, "All you need is a new man in your life."

I left his office wondering how he could say such a thing. My sex life prior to the surgery had been fine. Why should I get a new man in my life, because "I" felt so entirely different? My mate had not changed, I had changed. I knew the problem was within me.

By now, another realization was dawning on me. As a result of my vagina being cut, not only was one whole side numb, I also had no control over the muscles on that side. Even if I regained my ability to feel sexual again, I knew this would have an impact on my sex life forever.

As more months passed, it became obvious that the endocrinologist's new hormone therapy was not lifting my depression. I found it increasingly difficult to go to work. My daily routine consisted of forcing myself out of bed, moving to the couch, and lying there all day watching television. Even reading, one of my passions, no longer interested me.

Wanting to do nothing but hibernate, I found myself refusing all invitations to socialize. My lifelong friends, whom I had loved dearly, became an irritation to me. Never having felt like this before, I knew this depression was different. It felt like a chemical change, one over which I had no control, and nothing I did made any difference. I seemed to be caught in a downward spiral, falling deeper and deeper into a black hole, with no ability to climb out. After a year and a half, the doctors gave up on me. Repeatedly, their only answer was, "It must all be in your head. You really need to see a psychiatrist."

On one of my lethargic days of lying on the couch, I watched *The Phil Donahue Show*. His featured guest was a female gynecologist who described the symptoms of the hormone loss that can result from hysterectomies and oophorectomies. As the list of symptoms scrolled down the screen, realization dawned on me that almost every symptom matched what I had felt ever since my surgery. I could barely contain my excitement. At last, there might be someone who understood what I was going through. If other women were also experiencing these symptoms, maybe there was some hope after all. I knew I had to see her, and would have traveled anywhere to do so, but fortunately her office was only an hour's drive from my home.

Three weeks later, when I dragged myself into her office, she was not at all surprised at my description of what life had been like since my hysterectomy. Informing me that the amount of testosterone produced by the ovaries differs with every woman, it was her guess that I had been a high testosterone producer, and that I was feeling that loss even more than the estrogen loss. When I told her about my allergic reaction to the testosterone I had received, she explained that testosterone shots must be combined with estrogen to prevent women from reacting to the testosterone. Additionally, with my estrogen level still well below normal, she said I obviously was not absorbing the oral estrogen.

Next she asked if my blood pressure had always been high.

I explained that on my first visit to the surgeon after my hysterectomy, I was shocked when he warned me that my blood pressure was "dangerously high." At that time I told him, "I have never had high blood pressure. It has always been so low doctors and nurses consistently remarked how lucky I was to have such great blood pressure. How could I have suddenly developed high blood pressure?" The surgeon's only answer was, "I do not know why, but from now on we need to monitor you closely."

When I relayed this background history to the doctor, her reply sent me reeling. She explained, "High blood pressure is not uncommon after a hysterectomy. The uterus secretes a chemical that is involved in blood pressure regulation, and its loss is probably responsible for your present high blood pressure." This answer finally clarified what had been mystifying me since my surgery.

Before leaving her office, I received a shot of testosterone combined with estrogen, as well as a shot of vitamin B complex. In addition, she also prescribed a dietary supplement of amino acids.

Returning to my car, I felt like I was walking on air. At last, a doctor understood what I had been experiencing. In addition, her answers made logical sense, based upon the fact that my body was missing pieces of it's complex interdependent chemical structure. Driving home, even with the discouraging news about my high blood pressure, I felt the first hope I had known since my hysterectomy.

Hope, because this doctor had treated and helped many women who experienced what I was going through.

Hope, because she said she would not give up until she found the right combination of hormones to alleviate my symptoms.

Over the next several months, in her attempt to restore me to a level that felt as close to "normal" for me as possible, the doctor tried varying levels of hormones, as well as different methods of delivering them into my body. At first, nothing worked consistently. Oral estrogen was ruled out because I was not absorbing it. Skin patches did not work well, either. Up to this point, weekly shots worked the best. They made me feel more energetic, less depressed, and even produced days when I felt like my old self again. However, the shots were logistically impractical because the weekly trips to the doctor's office disrupted the better part of a work day.

By now, three years had gone by since my surgery; three years of living in hell. I needed to find a consistent, long-term hormone replacement that would relieve my symptoms, and allow me to work full time. As a last resort, the doctor tried using experimental hormone pellet implants. These tiny pellets, impregnated with estrogen or testosterone, are inserted into the fatty tissue of the buttocks or abdomen. Their gradual assimilation makes this form of replacement as much like a woman's natural ovary, as is artificially possible. The additional benefit of lasting anywhere from three to six months, also eliminates the inconvenience of weekly shots.

After having the estrogen and testosterone pellets implanted, I went home and prayed. My bottom was sore and I had to be careful how I sat, but by this time I was willing to try anything.

I expected and hoped for the same immediate results like I had felt from the shots, but that did not happen. One day went by, then two. No change. Then day three and four, no change. I was becoming discouraged. Since so many things had not helped up to this point, it was hard to believe that such tiny pellets could work. Incredibly, on day seven, I noticed a difference. Then day eight . . . better; day nine . . . even better. I felt lighter and slightly happier. Could it be? Would I finally be helped? Was it possible to feel like I had before the surgery?

At the end of two weeks, A MIRACLE occurred.

I felt like ME, whole again.

I was overjoyed. It was fun to smile and really mean it. It was great to be on top of the ground, instead of down in the bottom of a dark pit with sides too steep to climb out.

As I returned to the world of the living, I started sharing what my life had been like over the past three years. When people heard my story, they told me of other hysterectomized women who were experiencing the same deep, debilitating depression, and inability to get out of the house. In their concern, they asked me to contact their friends and convey to them how proper hormone replacement therapy was helping me.

As I met with these women, and listened to their descriptions of what their lives had been like since their surgery, I found many whose experiences were similar to mine. Several of them still had no relief from acute abdominal pain, and many shared their mutual frustration over a lack of sex drive. In addition, I discovered my consequences were not the only devastating conditions a hysterectomy can create. These women talked of thyroid dysfunction, and inability to control their weight. They spoke of additional surgeries being required to unblock intestinal obstructions created by adhesions from the scar. For some, intercourse had also become a physically painful experience, due to the anatomical changes created by the surgery. Others experienced hip damage, so severe that just the simple act of walking had become excruciatingly painful.

Hearing about these new problems prompted me to conduct a broader search in the medical libraries on the potential consequences of hysterectomies. Shock filled me as I began to uncover that everything we were experiencing had appeared in medical journals for almost a half a century. My horror continued to grow as I found 1,000's of articles all verifying what these women were telling me. Our symptoms were not just in our heads. We did not need psychiatrists as the doctors recommended—when out of frustration they did not know what else to do.

Based on this information, I filed a complaint with the California Medical Board. After months of waiting, I only received the following brief written response:

> "After our review of your file, we found that the doctor
> followed standard medical practice in performing
> your surgery. There is nothing to investigate.
> THE CASE IS CLOSED."

How could "standard medical practice" destroy a woman's quality of life for three years?

After going through such horrible grief myself, I wanted to warn other women, hoping to save them from blindly accepting "standard medical practice." I also knew I had to bring to the awareness of those who have had surgery that they need to take extra care of their bodies for the rest of their lives. The following chapters will clearly demonstrate: women's ovaries, uteruses, and cervixes are not "useless" after childbearing years, and that removal of their finely tuned chemical plants, nature so brilliantly provides, has the potential to create both immediate, and life-long devastating consequences. In order to make a truly informed choice, women deserve to be educated about all the repercussions which can arise from hysterectomies. Since the surgery is irreversible, the discussions about all the potentialities need to take place prior to surgery, not afterwards.

My now-grown daughter was nine at the time of my hysterectomy. When she recently shared with me how she felt during those black years following my surgery, I knew I had no other choice but to write this book. I did not want any other mother to hear her child say:

"When you came home from the hospital,
you weren't 'my Mom' anymore.
All I could think of was,
I wish I had my Mommy back."

2

Morbidity and Mortality:
Yes, You CAN DIE from the Surgery

Over the last 33 years between 20,000 to 40,000 women have died as a result of having a hysterectomy. The tragedy is, only 10% of them were facing any life-threatening condition prior to their surgery. This is only the beginning of the damage hysterectomies have created during their 100-year history.

How have we allowed this surgery to cause so much harm? To begin to understand, we need to look at the word itself.

Origin Of The Word: Hysterectomy

The origin of the word hysterectomy shows how little a woman's uterus has been valued, throughout almost the entire history of mankind. If we apply standard medical terminology (e.g., removal of the appendix is called an "appendectomy"), then removal of the uterus should be termed a "uterectomy." To find out why we use the term "hysterectomy" instead, we have to go back to the early Greeks. "Hyster", "hystera", and "hystero" stem from the Greek word meaning loss of emotional stability, and subject to fits of crying and laughing.[3] The Greeks, believing the uterus was the source of women's emotionality, concluded that it caused hysteria. Even though this outdated Greek notion developed during a time when little was known about how the human body functions, we, in the 20th century, still use a nomenclature which arose from this misconception. Understanding the role that this historic concept has had in shaping our attitudes about one of women's most important organs, helps explain why it has been so easy to convince women that removal of their uterus is not only necessary, but beneficial as well.

Even though the terminology is ancient in origin, hysterectomies are a relatively new phenomenon on the scene of mankind. Some of the first hysterectomies were performed in the late 1800's to save women from obvious life-threatening gynecological conditions, such as a gangrenous uterus. With the advent of modern antiseptic and anesthetic techniques, the practice started to take hold in the early 1900s. When the mortality (death) rate dropped down to 3%, doctors heralded hysterectomies as a great advancement in medicine, and began performing them on a routine basis in the 1930s.[4]

As surgical skills increased, they soon became the answer for many reproductive organ problems, gaining popularity so rapidly in the United States, that by the 1950s, hundreds of thousands were being performed every year. The rate continued to grow in record numbers, burgeoning to a peak of 725,000 in 1975.[5] This phenomenal rate finally stabilized, but still over 550,000 women undergo hysterectomies every year, making it second only to cesarean sections in numbers of operations performed in the United States.[6] In a little over 30 years, this incredibly high volume of surgeries has resulted in over 20 million women in America having their reproductive organs removed.[7]

Though the first hysterectomies were implemented to save women's lives, now only 10% are the result of cancer, and less than 1% for obstetrical emergencies.[8] The other, approximately 89%, are classified as "elective" surgery, and are performed for conditions that are not life-threatening.

Mortality

When starting the research for this book, the first thing that shocked me was the mortality (death rate) connected to the surgical removal of the uterus, alone. In modernized countries, study after study confirms the death rate, in the women who are not facing any life-threatening condition, is between 0.1 and 0.2%.[9] The medical community concludes that, since this rate is so low, hysterectomies are classified as a safe procedure to consider for a patient. True, it does sound low, but when multiplied by the over 20 million performed in America just since 1965, it translates into the staggering numbers, highlighted earlier in the chapter, of 20,000 to 40,000 women losing their lives as a result of this surgery.

The causes of death, including hemorrhage, cardiac arrest, heart attack, stroke, peritonitis, septicemia, pulmonary embolism, and bowel obstruction, are the direct result of the surgical procedure.[10] Articles even warn doctors: "Although overall hysterectomy is a safe operation when performed for the right indications, it must be remembered that it is a major procedure, and deep vein thrombosis (blood clots) and pulmonary embolism (blood clot or air in blood vessels in lung) can be significant causes of post-operative morbidity (complications) and mortality (death)."[11] One article concluded: "Early post-operative mortality (within 30 days of admission) appears to be low (16.1 per 10,000) and, compared to other surgical operations, it seems warranted to classify hysterectomy as a 'safe intervention'. However, it should be noted that these results (deaths) originate from patients who did not have diagnosed cancer and who had no major co-surgery (performed at the same time)." "Seen in this context it is necessary to take into consideration the risk of early post-operative death when choosing between surgical and other methods of treatment."[12]

Recognition of this is imperative, especially when the majority of hysterectomies (58.6%) are performed on women who are under the age of 45.[13] This means many women are struck down in the prime of their lives, and may even still have children at home.

Short-term Morbidity

After surviving the surgery, the next factor women need to be aware of is the immediate "short-term morbidity." Morbidity is defined as, anything that requires physician intervention, indicating concern for the patient's well-being. The morbidity rate connected to hysterectomies, even in countries using modern westernized techniques, is between 20 and 53%, depending on the type of procedure performed (e.g., vaginal vs. abdominal, etc.).[14]

Some of the complications, such as the average of 30% who experience serious infections, account for only short-term discomfort due to the availability of antibiotics.[15] However, this leads to the increased use of these drugs, helping to create more antibiotic-resistant bacteria.

Other surgical complications often have to be corrected, requiring extended hospital time, or additional surgery. The types of problems created are itemized below. The table shows the percentages, as well as the actual numbers of women affected, based on the 20 million hysterectomies performed since 1965.

Complication[16]	Percentage Of Women Affected	Total Affected Based On 20 Million
Additional surgical procedure to repair damage to bowel & bladder:	2.7%	.5 Million
Bladder and urination problems:	22.9%	4.6 Million
Injury to leg nerve:	11.6%	2.3 Million
Irritable bowel syndrome		
Increased symptoms:	20.0%	4.0 Million
New symptoms:	9.0%	1.8 Million
Longer hospital stay:	19.5%	3.9 Million
Need additional specialist:	9.1%	1.8 Million
Admitted to ICU:	3.6%	.7 Million
Hemorrhage requiring transfusion:	9.0%	1.8 Million
Readmitted to hospital:	2.3%	.5 Million

These new difficulties, as well as the additional health care costs, are created by what has been termed a "simple female procedure." This surgery's impact to our medical system is further evidenced by the statistics that 16 to 67% of all "intestinal obstruction" surgeries are the result of women having had previous abdominal hysterectomies.[17] This, in itself, is a life-threatening condition, since one of the studies also revealed that 5% of the patients died as a direct result of the bowel obstruction.[18]

In analyzing whether the complications are worth it, one study stated: "From the patient's point of view, it is worth noting that, on average, even after a 'simple' hysterectomy about one out of ten women encounters a readmission due to complications within the two years following operation." "Seen from society's point of view, it is important to acknowledge that a high volume enterprise such as hysterectomy is followed by a substantial amount

of hospital admissions with more or less related complications."
"When considering the foreseeable benefit from surgical removal
of the uterus the patient deserves information about the risk of
later complications such as infections and bleeding."[19]

Long-term Morbidity

The immediate deaths and short-term consequences,
tragic and costly as they are, are really only the beginning of the
detrimental changes created by hysterectomies. Since they are
silent and insidious, it is the long-term consequences that need to
be brought to the awareness, of not only women, but to our whole
society, as well.

Doctors gain consent to remove women's ovaries by placing
fear in them about the silence of ovarian cancer, and how it is too
late when the symptoms appear. Women are made to feel
confident, that by cutting out the "potential" of cancer at the same
time as their female problem, they will be free from disease and
danger, now, and in the future.

The truth is, removing these vital organs, and the chemicals
they produce, leads to other seemingly unrelated physical and
emotional consequences.[20] Unsuspectingly, women are left facing
new disease-states, many of which are life-threatening. They may
no longer be facing the risk of one of the 3 cancers (uterine,
ovarian, and cervical), which combined result in 24,000 deaths
each year.[21] The loss of these vital organs, however, catapults
women into a much higher risk for cardiovascular disease, stroke,
and osteoporosis, which combined kill approximately 500,000
women a year in the United States.[22]

If hysterectomies produced a 100% cure for women, then
maybe some of the complications and long-term consequences
might warrant taking these risks, but sadly, this is not the case.

Follow-up surveys, which ask women whether their surgery was beneficial or harmful, show as many as 59% respond that either their symptoms were made worse, or they now were experiencing new ones.[23]

Statistics like these make it difficult to comprehend why hysterectomies are still performed in such record numbers. It becomes even more difficult to understand, when a study comparing surgical interventions for conditions like benign ovarian cysts, proved that if a hysterectomy was performed at the same time, women developed 5 times more complications, when compared to those who did not have their uterus removed.[24] These complications included wound infections, ureteral injury, urinary tract infections, bowel obstruction, blood clots, blood transfusions due to more than double the blood loss, and death.[25]

Practice Worldwide

One reason I consented to the surgery was due to the fact that hysterectomies are such an accepted, commonplace practice here in America. Additionally, the second opinion I had sought, agreed that my only option was surgery. It never occurred to me that other options might be available, or that other countries could have different ways of treating female problems.

One day, while getting my weekly hormone shot, I noticed the assisting nurse was from Israel. On the previous night's news program, they had shown Israeli women being fired upon in their Kibbutz'. As I watched, I thought, if those women feel like I do, they would not have the energy to fight back, and they would probably just roll over and allow themselves to be killed. So, hoping that doctors in Israel might have a solution for what I was going through, I asked the nurse how they help women through the aftermath of hysterectomies in Israel. I had a difficult time comprehending her answer. It was simply, "We don't do them. They are not a commonplace practice in Israel." With all the suffering I had been through, this made a great deal of sense to me, and spurred me on to researching hysterectomies in other countries.

Upon investigating the practices and rates worldwide, there are many similarities, but also striking differences. One of the biggest differences is found in the rates performed in the United States compared to other countries of the world. In the early 1970s, Australia's rate of 379 hysterectomies per 100,000 women was less than half the rate of the 830 per 100,000 in the United States.[26] Even though the rate in America began declining, many more were still being performed than in other countries, with an average of 587 compared to 348 per 100,000 in Finland, between 1987 and 1989.[27]

Why has there been such an exponential growth rate in America compared to other modernized nations? What makes the difference? Are women really that different worldwide? No, they are not. The difference is in America's acceptance of hysterectomy as the answer for almost any female condition, as well as a lack of understanding surrounding the many roles the uterus and ovaries play.

Worldwide, even though the practice is not as common, the overwhelming majority of hysterectomies are also elective, and performed for non-life-threatening conditions. The most frequent reason is fibroid tumors (leiomyomata, or myoma: benign tumors of the muscle), while the second most common reason is either endometriosis (lining of uterus found in abnormal locations), recurrent uterine bleeding, or prolapsed uterus, depending on the country.[28]

The following table provides a brief overview of the differences between countries in:

(1)   percentage of women hysterectomized by age 60

(2)   percentage of ovaries taken at the same time as the uterus

(3)   percentage of hysterectomies performed for non-life-threatening conditions

(4)   percentage performed for fibroid tumors.

Table 2   **Hysterectomy Practices Worldwide**

	% Of Women Hyster. By Age 60	**% Ovaries Taken At Same Time**	**% Performed For Non-life-threatening Conditions**	**% Performed For Fibroid Tumors**
USA [29]	25%	52%	89%	33%
Australia [30]	25% [a]	20%		
Britain [31]	20% [b]	14%	94%	39%
Finland [32]	21%	24%	92%	51%
France [33]	9%			
Italy [34]		43%		74%
Pakistan [35]		28%	95%	44%
Thailand [36]		53%		48%

Note: Data were not available for all items.
(a) Age mid-50's
(b) Age 55

This information clearly indicates whether a woman loses her uterus, or ovaries, or both, depends greatly upon the country in which she lives. With statistics showing such a disparity in usage, it behooves all of us to take a closer look at whether this surgery is really necessary.

3

The Ovaries:
Finely Tuned, ESSENTIAL, Chemical Manufacturing Plants

Throughout this century, several major misconceptions surrounding the ovaries have been allowed to shape our present gynecological therapeutic practices. They are: *The ovaries shut down at menopause,* and *The only function of the ovaries is childbearing.* Belief in these notions has resulted in the establishment of the current philosophy: *The prophylactic (preventive) removal of ovaries is justified, because it decreases the risk of cancer.* This conclusion, even though based on erroneous beliefs, has led to the removal of healthy ovaries becoming standard medical practice for women over 40 when they undergo a hysterectomy.[37] As a result, 51% of all hysterectomized women in America lose their ovaries. This percentage dramatically increases to 76% for those between the ages of 45 and 54, leaving millions of women attempting to function without these essential organs.[38]

Why save the ovaries? To understand why, we need to analyze the beliefs surrounding their function based on the information that is available today.

First Misconception:
The Ovaries Shut Down At Menopause

Women, led to believe their ovaries will not be working in a few years anyway, have been urged to give up their "potentially" cancerous organs. In reality, however, ovaries continue working after menopause, and the products they keep producing are essential for a healthy functioning body.[39] Even though their estrogen production decreases, the amount they do contribute is still significant enough for researchers to conclude: "Therefore, the ovary must be considered a potential source of estradiol (estrogen) and testosterone in all postmenopausal women."[40]

Every day, the ovaries manufacture approximately 60 micrograms of testosterone.[41] In fact, their testosterone production becomes an increasingly more important portion of the total testosterone manufactured by a woman's body. After menopause, the amount generated by the body's non-ovarian sources declines, resulting in the ovaries' contribution of testosterone rising from 25 to 40% of the body's daily production.[42] This essential hormone is utilized by the body not only for sex drive, but for the critical roles of structural maintenance and repair. Equally important, it is converted elsewhere in the body into the estrogen women still need.[43]

Knowledge that the ovaries keep functioning well past menopause has been fully described in the medical literature for years. The following quotation, written in 1954, leaves little doubt about their continued contribution to a woman's feeling of well-being: "The common experience, however, of gynecologic surgeons in having their patients complain bitterly of a severe menopausal syndrome when ovaries have been removed years after cessation of menses, has established the fact of ovarian estrogenic function long after the menopause."[44]

Second Misconception:
The Only Function Of The Ovaries Is Childbearing

The ovaries are not just reproductive organs—they are the foundation of life. Not only does new life spring from them, they are also essential for the healthy continuation of life. Take away their valuable benefits and women no longer build strong bones and muscles, or manufacture healthy skin.[45] Their cardiovascular systems become stressed, as fat clogs their arteries, because the metabolism of the food they eat is altered in unhealthy ways.[46] Normal blood pressure becomes difficult to maintain.[47] Emotional stability, energy level, well-being, and appetite are affected, due to alteration of the chemicals in the brain.[48] In addition to all of this, the ability to respond sexually can be diminished.[49]

These conditions start appearing after the loss of ovarian function, because the many vital chemicals they manufacture are involved in every aspect of our bodily functions. Scientifically, some of them have been known for years (e.g., estrogen, testosterone, and progesterone), but many ovarian products, as well as their roles, still remain to be identified.[50]

Third Misconception:
The Prophylactic Removal Of Ovaries Is Justified, Because It Decreases The Risk Of Cancer

The fear of cancer, combined with belief in the first two misconceptions, has allowed another myth to take hold: *Removal of healthy ovaries is not only necessary, but beneficial as well.*

However, studies reveal doubts about the benefits of this procedure when they state: "In weighing all of these facts it seems that the best we could accomplish would be the prevention of subsequent ovarian cancer in 3 women out of every 10,000 hysterectomies."[51] This number is for development of the cancer only, not death from it. When the death rate from simple hysterectomies is 1 to 2 per every 10,000 operations, the practice of both hysterectomy, along with prophylactic removal of ovaries, appears to become even more senseless!

Tragically, the incredible irony surrounding this practice is shown by many studies which reach the same conclusion: ovaries that are left in place during a hysterectomy undergo cancerous changes less often than in the population as a whole.[52] In other words, the evidence indicates that having a hysterectomy decreases a woman's chance of developing cancer in ovaries which are left intact during surgery.[53] This reduction is from its already low 1.8% risk over a woman's lifetime.[54] Even though some studies indicate hysterectomy's protective effect decreases over time, others show that 25 years later the risk of cancer is still reduced.[55]

The following conclusion of a 1984 article continues to uncover why prophylactic removal is difficult to justify: "In the face of the exceedingly low incidence of ovarian cancer and its questionable prevention by prophylactic oophorectomy (ovaries removed), routine oophorectomy would deprive enormous numbers of women of the essential benefits afforded by these steroid-secreting (hormone producing) organs."[56]

The truth is: *The ovaries perform a multitude of functions.* Undergoing their prophylactic removal throws women's bodies into what has been coined "surgical menopause", because menopause starts immediately after surgery. Research proves: "Surgical menopause accelerates all the processes of natural menopause."[57] The effects on the body are tremendous. Articles conclude that it can be a difficult time for women, while their bodies are being thrust into the rapid adjustment required, as compared to the slow, gradual transition over the years that it takes for natural menopause. Not only is it an abrupt overnight change, but the complete loss of the chemicals, which would normally continue to be manufactured by menopausal ovaries, leads to more severe symptoms than women experience when they are allowed to go through menopause naturally.[58] These symptoms include greater cardiovascular damage and bone loss.[59]

The evidence available today all points to the fact that it is imperative to heed these words written by researchers in 1984: "Because oophorectomy has such profound influences at every age, particularly its devastating relation to osteoporosis, and because there are no meaningful data in the literature to support the value of routine oophorectomy, we suggest that oophorectomy only be performed when the ovaries are diseased."[60]

Fourth Misconception:
Ovaries Left Intact During A Hysterectomy Will Continue Optimal Functioning

Women who elect to save their ovaries, feeling confident they will be left with the protection these organs provide, need to be aware of another major myth: *Ovaries left intact during a hysterectomy will continue optimal functioning*. Sadly, saving the ovaries does NOT guarantee they will, and this assumption leaves many women in the dark about the potential post hysterectomy changes that can occur in their bodies.

Removal of just the uterus, alone, can result in ovarian failure. Research reveals as many as 20 to 44% of hysterectomized women may experience decreased ovarian function, or ovarian failure, as compared to 13% in women who have not had surgery.[61] One article, studying women undergoing hysterectomy for cervical cancer, stated that as long as 20% of the ovaries were going to shut down anyway, they should be taken at the same time as the uterus.[62] This recommendation, published in 1993, was predicated on a hypothetical cost comparison of one combined surgery (ovaries and uterus removed), versus two operations, in the event there was a future problem with the ovaries. Based on this, they concluded that: ". . . the cost of preserving the ovaries may exceed that of removing them."[63] Yet, the actual risk of a second operation being required is only between 3.5 and 8%.[64]

Even when both ovaries are preserved, many studies demonstrate that young hysterectomized women experience the following abnormal hormonal and menopausal symptoms:

1.   23% show increased follicle stimulating hormone (FSH) levels, which is indicative of decreased ovarian function.[65]

2.   they have significantly lower bone densities.[66]

3.   39% demonstrate deficient progesterone levels one month following surgery. When retested 6 months after surgery, 40% of these patients still had not regained normal functioning.[67]

Additional proof of decreased ovarian function is provided in a large study of approximately 1,000 hysterectomized women, who were compared to over 5,000 non-hysterectomized women. Even though they still had their ovaries, the hysterectomized women all showed postmenopausal signs and complaints. These symptoms were so prevalent, the study ended with a warning to physicians to be alert to typical menopausal complaints in hysterectomized women, especially in young women, even when their ovaries have been preserved. As a group, they show a greater incidence rate in all the disease states associated with menopause, including osteoporosis, cardiovascular disease, osteoarthritis, depression, and sexual problems.[68]

When only one ovary is left, there is an even greater possibility that it will shut down. This result is so common, one research article concluded with: "The fact that one-third of the patients undergoing USO (one ovary removed) will develop ovarian dysfunction raises the question whether there is a place for this procedure."[69]

These results would not occur if the preserved ovaries were still functioning.[70] Moreover, they prove that even when their ovaries are conserved women cannot know in advance whether, or not, they will be thrown into surgical menopause. It is a GAMBLE.

Uterus Removal Leads To Early Menopause

Unfortunately, even the women who are lucky enough to have their ovaries remain functional, wind up entering menopause years earlier than their non-surgical counterparts.[71] As long ago as 1932, a study looking into this question found the frequency of menopausal symptoms in women under 40 to be eight times greater than in those who did not undergo a hysterectomy, with the symptoms occurring within 2 years of the operation in 92% of these women.[72] Overall, as many as 44% of hysterectomized women enter menopause by the age of 45, versus only 13% of women who never had surgery.[73]

Though numerous articles prove a direct relationship exists between hysterectomy and early menopause, very few women are informed of this potential.[74] As a result, when women start developing menopausal symptoms after a hysterectomy, they do not understand what is happening in their bodies, and may not get the help they need.

Why does a premature shut down occur immediately in some women and not in others? One possible reason is that chemicals secreted by the uterus are part of a feedback loop that stimulates the ovaries.[75] Disruption of this feedback could also explain why tubal ligations can lead to many symptoms of hormone disruption, including menstrual disturbances and abnormal cycles.[76]

A second possible reason, damage during surgery, was being theorized as early as 1935. At the time, doctors stated: "If this fact be true, it suggests that hysterectomy with ovarian conservation brings about menopausal symptoms through injuring the ovarian blood supply rather than through the absence of the uterus per se."[77]

Today's research confirms that ovaries can, indeed, be damaged by disruption to the blood vessels or the nerves leading to them. Every part of the body is dependent on a full supply of blood and nerves. If either of these are cut off to an arm or a leg, the limb will become useless and wither. This is easy to see because it is external, while the internal changes resulting from a hysterectomy are not so recognizable. One study, looking into this potentiality, found that during surgery the blood flow through the ovaries can be reduced by 52 to 89% in premenopausal women.[78] Even though it is temporary, this acute reduction of blood could lead to impaired functioning of the ovaries, which may not be recognized until menopausal symptoms surface.

Not only has research proved that the ovaries can be subjected to decreased blood flow during surgery, it has also established that every body is unique. Utilizing arteriography methods (artery x-rays) to look at normal blood flow to the ovaries, researchers concluded: "The general opinion is that the uterine artery supplies the medial (middle) half of the ovary and the medial two-thirds of the (fallopian) tube, the rest of their blood supply coming from the ovarian artery. The distribution of these arteries, however, shows great variation. In extreme cases either artery alone (uterine or ovarian) may supply the entire tube and ovary." "All possibilities may occur, ranging from cases in which the ovarian artery supplies the entire (fallopian) tube and ovary to cases in which the blood supply of these organs is solely derived from the uterine artery."[79] Based on these findings, those women whose uterine artery solely supplies their ovaries may be the ones who experience immediate menopause. Additionally, if half of the ovaries' blood supply comes from the uterine arteries, disruption of this source could account for the earlier onset of menopause created by hysterectomies.

This randomness, in whether the blood supply is temporarily or permanently cut off, helps account for the wide range of women's reactions to surgery. There is no way to detect the extent of this phenomenon until after surgery. A doctor will have one patient who does well, while another will start experiencing all the symptoms of menopause, or depression, due to the sudden lack of hormones her body had been so eloquently producing for her. Believing he didn't do anything differently, the doctor may question the validity of her symptoms.

The Total Functions Of The Ovary Are Still Unknown

The medical community is still very much in the dark as to the total physiological functioning of the ovary, either premenopausal or postmenopausal.[80] Investigators even conclude that there is a lack of both epidemiological investigations of hysterectomized versus non-hysterectomized women, as well as a poverty of knowledge about roles the ovaries continue to play throughout women's lives coming from the laboratories.[81] As a result, researchers are just now identifying some of the chemicals which are lost due to the removal of childbearing organs. These chemicals are so new, they do not have names yet. Letters and numbers are assigned to them, while scientists attempt to classify them. However, this is only one part of the puzzle. The roles they perform are still part of the mystery under investigation. How can doctors artificially replace something when they have no idea what it is, what it does, how much is needed, or when it is needed. It can't be done.

In reality, after almost a century of removing these organs by the millions, medical science is only beginning to piece together the complex inter-relationship these essential hormone and chemical manufacturing organs have with the rest of the body.[82] There are still many areas remaining to be explored and clarified as to how the ovaries function throughout a woman's life. Until more is understood, "standard medical practice" should not mean removing healthy organs, whose entire functions remain unknown, and therefore cannot possibly be replaced.

4

The Cervix IS Important:
Why It Should Be Preserved

In America, hysterectomy has come to mean the removal of the cervix along with the uterus, 99% of the time.[83] Women have not been informed that losing their cervix during surgery is optional. Like millions of women, I was lured into the false web of belief that our cervixes are another relatively unimportant part of our anatomy. However, while conducting research for this book, the following statements from two articles caught my attention.

1)   "The subtotal, cervix-sparing hysterectomy lost favor in this country (USA) in the early 1960s for reasons relating to prevention of cervical cancer and because 'the cervix doesn't contribute to sexual satisfaction anyway,' an axiom often repeated to medical students at the time. While cancer prevention is laudable, the actual risk (of cervical cancer) is low, and screening technologies and the naturally slow course of the disease are such that many today would reconsider the prophylactic removal of the cervix."[84]

2)   "It is concluded that the risk of developing carcinoma (cancer) of the cervical stump is low, and no longer a weighty indication for the total (removal of both uterus and cervix) in preference

to the supravaginal hysterectomy as long as subsequent screening (Pap smears) of the cervix is performed."[85]

Up to this point, having never thought much about my cervix, or its function, the fact that I lost it through surgery had not meant much to me. Therefore, I was not looking for information about the cervix, or its function, and had no plans to include a chapter on it in this book. Since hysterectomy is generally referred to as the taking of the uterus and cervix as one unit, and because my doctor never mentioned that it was elective, I assumed it to be a necessary part of the procedure. Now, however, after reading these two statements, questions plagued my mind. What is a "subtotal" or "supravaginal" hysterectomy? Is there really a choice as to how a uterus is removed, and what must be taken with it? Has fear of cancer been the only reason for the removal of the cervix at the same time as the uterus?

Pulling out my medical dictionary and textbooks, I looked up these procedures. The medical dictionary indicates that a hysterectomy does not have to include the removal of the cervix. It defines hysterectomy as: "Total or partial surgical removal of the uterus."[86] In other words, "total" hysterectomy means, the uterus and cervix are both removed at the time of surgery. While "partial", "supravaginal" (supracervical), or "subtotal" hysterectomy means only the uterus is removed, leaving the cervix in place.

As I kept exploring, I was amazed to find that the *National Cancer Institute's (NCI)* information pamphlet, *What You Need To Know About Cancer Of The Uterus,* defines hysterectomy as: "An operation that removes the uterus and cervix."[87] Anyone reading this definition would believe that hysterectomy means the cervix has to be removed with the uterus. This is just one example of how women in America are not presented with complete information about the choices they have regarding their bodies. We believe we can trust that we are receiving the information we need to help us make informed health decisions. If this is so, then why did it take 8 years for me to uncover that I had a choice about saving my cervix?

Further research confirmed that the "standard medical practice" of taking a woman's cervix at the same time as the uterus is optional. It was originally adopted to prevent the "possibility" of future cervical cancer, not because the cervix is so intricately connected with the uterus that it has to be removed at the same time. Doctors have justified the removal of the cervix during a hysterectomy by stating they are saving women from being one of the 6,000 women who die each year from cervical cancer.

In the 1960s, when doctors were routinely removing women's cervixes, the rate for the potential of developing cervical cancer was 30.8, with a death rate of 10.6 per 100,000 women.[88] If in 1965, 100% of the American doctors adopted this prevention plan, then the 384,000 women hysterectomized for non-cancerous reasons lost their cervixes, when 118 of them were actually facing the possibility of developing cervical cancer, and only 41 faced dying from it.[89]

The good news is that over the 24 year period between 1965 and 1988, both the incidence, as well as the death rate, have been cut by more than half. The potential of developing cervical cancer fell to 8.6, with the risk of dying from it decreasing to 4.3 per 100,000.[90] Today, however, this low rate means that of the approximately 500,000 hysterectomies performed each year for non-life-threatening conditions, only 43 of the women even face the potential of developing cervical cancer, with only 22 having the possibility of dying from it. Yet, between 300 to 1,000 women die every year from their hysterectomy surgery, alone.[91] We have all heard the phrase, "The cure is worse than the disease." In this case, it definitely is.

Doctors may argue that the decrease in the cervical cancer death rate is due to their removing the potentially cancerous cervixes. However, this is not the case. The U.S. Centers for Disease Control (CDC) reports that the more than 50% drop reflects only non-hysterectomized women, and credits the Pap test, not hysterectomies, for the decline.[92]

Studies, dating as far back as 1935, provide the ultimate proof that removing women's cervixes in fear of potential cancer is totally unfounded. They reveal that the incidence of cancer developing in the remaining cervical stump was only 1.76% back then.[93] Even in the face of this low rate, the prophylactic removal was so championed that in 1969 one doctor editorialized: "Today, if the cervix is permitted to remain, the gynecologist must justify his failure to remove it."[94]

Today, with the decline in the cervical cancer rate, combined with the widespread use of Pap tests, this practice makes even less sense; particularly so, when the incidence of cervical cancer developing in the remaining stump is now only 0.1%, or nearly a zero risk.[95]

In the United States, the shift to routinely removing the cervix occurred by 1955. It is estimated by that time, 99.5% of the hysterectomies included the cervix.[96] In Mexico, as in the United States, close to 100% of their hysterectomies include the cervix.[97] This practice, however, differs greatly throughout the world. For example, in Sweden the rate is 79%, whereas China is the most conservative, removing them only 18% of the time.[98]

Saving The Cervix

Even with my medical background and all my years of research, I never realized the many functions the cervix performs functions that women are not aware of until they have lost them, and then it is too late.

Why save the cervix? To begin with, when the cervix is saved, the surgical trauma is greatly reduced, resulting in fewer complications and more women obtaining relief from their symptoms.

1.   Fewer Complications

In the initial surgery alone, conserving the cervix produces fewer complications, and results in a much shorter recovery time.[99] Table 3 below compares some of the factors involved.

Table 3
Comparative Surgical Outcomes—Laparoscopic [a] Hysterectomy

Conditions	Total [b]	Vs.	Subtotal [c]
Blood Loss	250		50 cc
Hospital Stay	37		18 Hours
Ability to Return to Work	22		7 Days
Return to Normal Activity	14		3 Days

Notes:
(a) Scope used to view interior of abdomen.
(b) Uterus and cervix taken (vaginal)
(c) Cervix saved (abdominal)

Source: Lyons TL. Laparoscopic supracervical hysterectomy: A comparison of morbidity and mortality results with laparoscopically assisted vaginal hysterectomy. *Jour Reproductive Med.* 1993 Oct. 38(10):763-7.

2. Greater Relief From Symptoms

A higher percentage of women experience relief from their pre-hysterectomy symptoms when their cervixes were saved. Tables 4 and 5 clearly show this by comparing the percentage of women who experience relief from their symptoms one year after surgery, depending on whether the cervix was removed or saved.

Percentage of Women Experiencing Symptoms

Table 4 **Cervix Removed**

Condition	Experiencing Symptoms Prior To Surgery	Experiencing Symptoms 1 Year After Surgery	% Of Women Helped
Bladder pressure	33.3%	9.6%	**71%**
Residual urine pressure	28.6%	22.1%	**23%**
Incontinence	36.2%	28.8%	**20%**

Table 5 **Cervix Saved**

Condition	Experiencing Symptoms Prior To Surgery	Experiencing Symptoms 1 Year After Surgery	% Of Women Helped
Bladder pressure	38.3%	10.3%	**73%**
Residual urine pressure	35.5%	10.3%	**71%**
Incontinence	47.7%	22.6%	**53%**

Source: Kilkku P. Supravaginal uterine amputation versus hysterectomy with reference to subjective bladder symptoms and incontinence. *Acta Obstet Gynecol Scand.* 1985. 64:375-9.

As indicated in Table 4, only 71%, 23%, or 20% of the women who lost their cervix experienced relief from their symptoms. When their cervixes were spared (Table 5), the numbers of women gaining relief for each of the three symptoms increased to 73%, 71%, and 53%, respectively—a dramatic difference. Women go into surgery expecting their symptoms to be alleviated, but these results prove that when their cervixes are removed, fewer women are helped.

3.   Long-term Consequences Of Cervical Removal

Even though the recovery from surgery is easier and a higher percentage of women experience relief from their symptoms, the most important reasons for saving the cervix are the long-term consequences. Once it is removed, loss of its many functions cannot be regained. The problems that can arise include:

A.   Loss Of Cervical Mucus

1.   A Bacteria Barricade

The mucus produced by the cervix has antibacterial properties enabling it to function as a barrier to bacteria and yeast. This action provides natural protection against upper genital tract infections.[100]

2.   Vital Chemicals

The cervix is not just a physical guard at the neck of women's wombs. The mucus it secretes is filled with abundant quantities of prostaglandins; chemicals known to have multiple effects on the nervous system, and on physiological functioning as well.[101] However, again, the tragedy is that medical science is only now beginning to identify them, and is a long way from understanding the important roles they play in the well-being of our bodies. It is difficult to comprehend how, in just the last 33 years, well over 20 million women have lost such vital chemicals, when today's research articles end with: "The biologic significance of these cervical mucus PGs (prostaglandins) is unknown."[102] In other words, studies have not uncovered what happens to the body when these prostaglandins are lost as a result of hysterectomies. Until more is known, their preservation becomes even more critical, since prostaglandins cannot be replaced.

B. **Nerve Loss And Structural Changes**

1. **Vaginal Prolapse**

Removing the cervix can result in the nerve and blood supply to the upper part of the vagina being cut off, as well as a greater disruption to the anatomy and supporting ligaments of the pelvic area.[103] This may create a susceptibility to degeneration, as well as a higher percentage of vaginal prolapse (a falling down or turning outward of vagina), which occurs from 0.1% to 18% of the time.[104]

2. **Bladder And Rectal Dysfunction**

There is a large nerve complex that connects to the ureters, bladder, rectum, uterus, and vagina. The lower portion of this complex, termed the Frankenhauser's plexus, can be damaged when the cervix is removed.[105] In addition, total hysterectomy may result in loss of the support for the bladder.[106] Either consequence can leave women with bladder or rectal dysfunction.[107]

3.   Decreased Ability To Enjoy Sex

Loss of the cervix contributes to this in several ways.

a.   Anatomical Changes
And Scar Tissue Formation.

When the cervix is removed, normal anatomy can be destroyed and scar tissue can form in the vagina.[108] This could lead to any number of problems, including either increased pain, or decreased feeling.

b.   Loss Of Nerve Complex

The cervix's intricate connection to the Frankenhauser's nerve complex, with its many nerve endings, makes the cervix sensitive to pressure.[109] The fact that a large portion of this nerve complex is lost when the cervix is removed, led one researcher to theorize: ". . . excision (removal) of the cervix is bound to have an adverse effect on sexual arousal and orgasm in women who previously experienced internal orgasm."[110]

Follow up studies show that as many as 10-50% of hysterectomized women complain that their sex life deteriorated after surgery.[111] The importance of the cervix's role in sexual satisfaction is emphasized by statements such as: "However, a few new studies indicate a reduced frequency of orgasm after the total hysterectomy compared with the supravaginal (cervix sparing) operation."[112]

One study investigating this phenomenon found that prior to surgery, 29% of the women reported they reached orgasm less than ¼ of the time. After surgery, this number increased to 47% in those women who had a total hysterectomy (cervix removed), versus an increase to 32% for the women whose cervixes were spared.[113]

Here again, due to the tremendous individual differences found between people, only a certain number of women report that pressure on the cervix is essential for them to obtain a fulfilling orgasm.[114] This helps add to the conflicting results from studies, and leaves doctors perplexed over the variable responses of their patients. Since it is difficult for a woman to understand, beforehand, exactly where her orgasm originates, she only realizes that the feeling is lost, afterwards, when nothing can be done to replace the nerves and tissue that were removed. Women deserve to be forewarned that they are gambling with their ability to respond sexually, and to be sexually fulfilled.

After reviewing the literature investigating the functions of the cervix, as well as the risks and benefits of its removal during a hysterectomy, one researcher concluded: "The cervix is not a useless organ; it should not be removed without a proper indication."[115]

These outcomes show that salvaging the cervix is of concern for women everywhere. In the 1950s, when doctors were making the decision to automatically remove this important organ, its many functions were not understood. In addition, the theory that its removal would reduce the risk of death from cervical cancer was not tested.

Today, the evidence is in. Mass removal of the cervix has not been responsible for reducing the risk of cervical cancer, while the loss of its benefits compromises both women's health, and the quality of their lives.

5

High Blood Pressure:
Unknown Risk

The mystery of how premenopausal hysterectomies lead to a 3-fold increase in cardiovascular disease begins to be revealed in this chapter.[116]

After surgery, I realized my newly acquired high blood pressure put me at risk for a stroke—a stroke that could kill me instantly. When this condition began, I still had an 11 year old daughter at home. Who would raise her if I died, or became paralyzed by a stroke?

These fears spurred me to start doing everything I could to bring my blood pressure under control. I joined a gym and worked out as though my life depended on it. It did! I tried all the recommended exercise routines for improving cardiac health. I used the cardiovascular machines for a full 30 minutes, at least 5 times a week. I lost 15 pounds, yet my blood pressure never budged. I continued to work out religiously, hoping against hope that my blood pressure would come down. It didn't. When my doctor recommended a "low salt" diet, I avoided salt at all cost, even refusing to eat in restaurants for months at a time. When the time spent exercising and maintaining a low-salt diet didn't work, I started trying everything else I read or heard about (e.g., garlic, cayenne, and evening primrose oil). Yet, nothing seemed to make any difference. My blood pressure still remained high!

After 5 years with no change, I realized I had only one choice left—to consider taking medication. There are several types available for high blood pressure, but each has its own varying degrees of side-effects. I spoke with people who had tried many of them before they found one their bodies could tolerate. Upon hearing all of their difficulties, however, I chose what I felt at the time to be the lesser of the two evils—to take no medication and just let my blood pressure remain high. At least, for now, I would not have to experience a medication's side-effects.

I went on with my life, resolving to keep doing all I could to help decrease the risk of stroke. I kept exercising regularly and maintained a low salt, low fat diet. Olives became an incredibly great treat four times a year.

Three more years went by. When a new job required traveling for weeks at a time, I was forced to eat restaurant food again, which limited my ability to regulate the amount of salt in my diet. In addition, while on one of my lengthy road trips, I became sick and began taking medications for a cold and severe cough. Not realizing that both medications increased blood pressure, I wound up in a hospital emergency room with dangerously high blood pressure, resulting in a $3,000 overnight hospital stay, plus time lost from work.

This emergency room episode made me realize that I had to try blood pressure medication. I actually had no choice because the cardiologist would not let me leave the hospital until my blood pressure was under control. Fortunately, the first one he prescribed brought it down within an hour and I felt fine. Feeling relieved, I chastised myself on the way home from the hospital for not trying medication sooner, and placing myself at high risk of a stroke for so many years.

After several weeks, though, I found it difficult to do anything requiring muscle exertion. I became exhausted trying to complete my routine workout at the gym. While traveling, the simple act of going up an incline at an airport left me breathless.

Concerned, I made an appointment with my primary care physician. She advised, "Let's wean you off the blood pressure medication. You don't want to stay on it, because it's not good for you in other ways." Unfortunately, even at only half dosage, my blood pressure shot back up to a dangerous range. Upon my return to the doctor, her words of warning were, "You can't stop the medication after all. You have to keep your blood pressure down." She prescribed a different class of medication, hoping it wouldn't create the exhausted effect I was, by then, continuously feeling.

As I gradually increased the dosage of the new medication, my muscles started hurting. After several weeks, the ends of every muscle hurt, including those is my lungs. Each breath was becoming agonizing, and I couldn't get through a night without waking up in pain. It never occurred to me to relate these effects to the medication until a friend asked, "What are you doing that's different?" I stopped the medication, and within a week the pain went away, but my blood pressure shot back up. Again, my doctor stressed, "You need medication. Your blood pressure must be controlled."

So which do I face? Do I put up with the side-effects of medications, or do I stop taking them? Do I go through life as a walking time bomb, wondering, what if I have a stroke? It's probably not IF, it's more likely, WHEN will I have a stroke? When I do, how bad will it be? Will I die? Will I be paralyzed? If I am paralyzed, how bad will it be? Will it be all on one side, or will it just impair my ability to speak? How long would it take me to recover? Who would pay for the care? Who would support my daughter and me?

Prior to surgery, I did not have to face any of these questions. Was the attempt to alleviate my pain and heavy bleeding worth risking death, or being paralyzed for the rest of my life? No, absolutely not! I did not understand why my doctor had not informed me of this potential consequence of losing my uterus.

When the program of diet and exercise did not lower my blood pressure, and the medications created such adverse effects, I knew there had to be more to the puzzling correlation between high blood pressure and hysterectomies. Since I had been on a satisfactory hormone replacement therapy (HRT) program of estrogen, progesterone, and testosterone during most of this struggle, I knew these were not the missing pieces.

So, back to the libraries once again. Here, words of warning about the life-threatening nature of high blood pressure jumped out at me from the medical journals. I found: "On average, when compared with people with controlled high blood pressure, people with uncontrolled high blood pressure are:

- ♥ 3 times more likely to develop coronary heart disease;
- ♥ 6 times more likely to develop congestive heart failure; and
- ♥ 7 times more likely to have a stroke."[117]

In addition, many studies confirmed my experience. After observing that a greater percentage of hysterectomized women suffer from high blood pressure, one group of researchers concluded: "The main finding of our study was that hysterectomy with ovarian preservation is associated with increased diastolic (minimum) blood pressure and the diagnosis of hypertension (high blood pressure)." They reached this conclusion when they found that 36% of hysterectomized women exhibit high blood pressure, compared to 21% in the population as a whole. When hysterectomy is combined with oophorectomy, the percentage becomes 44%—more than double the general population.[118]

Findings from this study also confirmed my lack of response to HRT. Whether they were taking HRT or not, 44% of oophorectomized women displayed high blood pressure, leaving them to struggle with this life-threatening condition for the rest of their lives. It is interesting to note, however, this study also found that the use of hormone replacement therapy did have a positive influence on blood pressure for women who had a hysterectomy only.[119] Conflicting results like these are what have led researchers to issue a warning that the blood pressure of women on any type of hormone therapy should be monitored.[120]

With research revealing that high blood pressure is the most important risk factor for coronary artery disease and stroke, it becomes vital to understand its link to hysterectomies.[121] In my desperation, I hoped I might find researchers who were not only studying the high blood pressure created by hysterectomies, but were attempting to isolate what life-sustaining chemicals are lost due to the operation.

My library search had begun by looking for the uterine chemicals the new gynecologist had mentioned. It did not take long, however, before I found many disturbing reasons why a woman's blood pressure is connected to chemicals found in the uterus, and the ovaries as well.

The rest of this chapter briefly covers some of the chemicals which are potentially lost, along with the influential functions they perform in the extremely complicated process of blood pressure regulation in the body.

Chemicals Of Both The Ovaries And Uterus

Renin And Angiotensin System

Renin and angiotensin are part of a complex hormone system that plays a primary role in maintaining normal blood pressure throughout the body. These hormones exert profound effects on blood pressure by affecting how much blood vessels constrict.[122] Originally, physiologists thought the hormones and chemicals involved with this system were produced only in the liver and kidneys, but it is now well established that they are also found in the uterus, as well as the ovaries and testicles.[123]

During pregnancy many women routinely maintain lower than normal blood pressure. Testing women's blood at this time reveals that the components of the renin-angiotensin system, as well as their activity, are increased 4-fold and more over normal values.[124] Since studies also verify that some of these chemicals originate directly from the ovaries, and that people with high blood pressure have 35% lower than normal levels, and whatever the ovary manufactures could be involved in providing this protection of lowered blood pressure body-wide.[125]

The Low Salt Diet Recommendation

The physiological importance of the renin-angiotensin system is illustrated by a recently completed study. For many years the medical community has recommended a low salt diet for everyone with high blood pressure. This recommendation came after seeing how salt, by itself, increased pressure on the blood vessels. They theorized that this would create high blood pressure. The one thing they neglected to look at, however, was whether low salt might be harmful to the body, as a whole. As a result, the findings of this study conflict with the widely held popular belief that a low salt diet is beneficial.

After following approximately 1,900 men over a three year period, the researchers found that those with the least amount of salt in their diet had the most deaths from heart attacks![126] Upon investigation, they realized no one had ever looked at the fact that decreased salt causes the kidneys to excrete the renin part of the renin-angiotensin system. Studies on high blood pressure patients reveal that salt deprivation leads to more than a doubling of prorenin (renin's precursor) and renin activity in the blood.[127] The increased renin results in the cascade of chemicals which ultimately causes constriction of the blood vessels.[128] When this action of renin is combined with any fat build-up in the arteries, the end result can be a heart attack.[129]

Doctors have advised people with high blood pressure to go on low salt diets for many years, without looking into whether it might kill them! This is exactly the same as advising women for almost a century to have hysterectomies, without looking into whether the surgery might result in other conditions, like high blood pressure, that could harm or eventually kill them, years later.

Chemicals Of The Ovaries

Substance P

Loss of the ovaries, or their function, may indirectly alter blood pressure by changing the concentration of other chemicals that do have a direct influence on blood pressure. Research is beginning to show this may be the case with a potent vasodilator called "substance P."[130] Research animals show that a loss of ovarian function results in reduced levels of substance P. They also reveal that as estrogen (17β-estradiol) concentrations rise, there is a parallel increase of substance P.[131] In addition to regulating the level of substance P, estrogen has also been shown to enhance the vasodilating action of this chemical in postmenopausal women.[132]

These recent findings have led some researchers to theorize that one of estrogen's beneficial actions is its influence on substance P.[133] If this is true, here is another way this ovarian hormone protects the cardiovascular systems of premenopausal women.

Serotonin

Serotonin influences many bodily functions. One area being intensely investigated is its variable interaction with blood platelets (clotting agents in the blood), which impacts the blood pressure in a subset of the population, especially as people age.[134] Alterations in this system also appear to be involved with the high blood pressure of pregnancy that can lead to eclampsia (convulsions).[135] Since both aging and pregnancy create these critical changes, the ovaries and uterus may play important roles in blood pressure—highlighting additional ways hysterectomies can result in the loss of the ability to maintain normal blood pressure.

Chemicals Of The Uterus

The uterus produces large quantities of chemicals called prostacyclin and prostaglandins.[136] I was amazed at the numerous studies examining their functions, indicating that this is a huge area of investigation. Researchers do not talk about just one prostaglandin, they discuss a very large complex of chemicals involved in a spectacular cascade, which causes a multitude of reactions to occur at any one time.

Prostacyclin acts as a potent vasodilator that relaxes arteries, and prostaglandins are involved in either constricting or relaxing artery walls.[137] With these types of actions, they can have very strong effects on blood pressure. So far, studies have concentrated on the roles they perform during pregnancy and labor. However, this is clearly a new area of research, with many more questions than there are answers. Investigators really don't know the total functions of any of these chemicals, or how their loss affects a woman throughout her life.

The Body's Automatic Checks And Balances

The human body is a wondrous maze of interwoven systems of checks and balances. While in a college Human Physiology class, I remember marveling so much at the amazing miracle of our bodies, that I decided to make medicine my career. An example of one of the "miracles" is our oxygenating system, which is constantly on auto pilot, insuring that sufficient oxygen gets to our tissues no matter how much is available in the air. When we are oxygen-deprived, such as climbing a mountain, 5 different physiological reactions take place. This is such a totally automatic response, we just take it for granted that our bodies will adapt, no matter what the surroundings.

When we go up in altitude, the drop in pressure of the oxygen gas in the air we breathe is detected by delicate sensor cells in the heart's aorta and the carotid (neck) arteries, producing the following incredible changes:[138]

1) Increased alveolar ventilation (increased exchange of oxygen and carbon dioxide in the lungs).

2)   Increased cardiac (heart) output.

3)   The kidneys increase their production of a hormone called erythropoietin, instructing the body to manufacture more of the oxygen carrying red blood cells, as well as more hemoglobin (that part of the red blood cell which carries the oxygen molecule).

4)   The plasma (which transports the red blood cells) decreases in volume, leaving more red blood cells per drop of blood (by volume). The end result is more oxygen available per drop of blood as it flows through the capillaries.

5)   The pH (acidity) in the blood stream changes. This increases the red blood cells' ability to give up the oxygen molecule it carries to the oxygen thirsty cells.

If all this did not take place immediately, automatically, and simultaneously, we could not function above 10,000 feet. Without all these backup and fail-safe insurances for our survival built into our awesome, intricately woven human bodies, we would not be able to fly, snow ski, or climb the Mt. Everests of the world. Our life expectancy would be very short, and we would not have the ability to inhabit the four corners of the earth.

Even knowing all this, and after more than 100 years of intensive study by the world's greatest respiratory physiologists, researchers state they still do not completely understand how the body automatically responds to the increased demand for oxygen.[139]

With so many safeguards protecting our ability to exist on this planet, it makes sense that nature also protects women during pregnancy, to assure their survival, the survival of their babies, and ultimately, the survival of the species. High blood pressure during pregnancy can lead to toxemia and death, for either the mother, or the baby, or both. Maintaining normal blood pressure is crucial for women at this time. Having the uterus, as well as the ovaries producing chemicals which influence blood pressure, follows right along with the marvelous ways our bodies have been designed to guarantee the miracle of life, itself.

When I discovered these important uterine and ovarian chemicals, my surgeon's postoperative words echoed in my head: "We believe the ovaries make about 13 different chemicals, although not all of them have been identified." Here was proof that this was true, not only for the ovaries, but for the uterus as well, since they produce chemicals that may affect both women's blood pressure and their nervous systems in ways that are still unexplored. Many studies are currently being conducted which are attempting to decipher their functions, but unfortunately, it could be that even in another 100 years, we still may not understand their total function, how they interact, or what effect they have on the rest of the body.

No wonder my blood pressure could not be regulated. I was missing valuable pieces of the jig-saw puzzle. Try to pick up a jig-saw puzzle with pieces of the puzzle missing-it falls apart. Hysterectomizing women strips away the checks and balances that maintain their life-preserving blood pressure regulation, leaving them facing this battle for the rest of their lives.

Our bodies are an incredible phenomenon of awesome efficiency. There is nothing produced that is not needed. If female reproductive organs manufacture chemicals, there must be a reason for them. Just because scientists have not identified or determined the functions of all these chemicals, it does not mean that they are expendable. If anything, when we have no idea how their loss impacts the entire body, the principles of "standard medical practice" should mandate even more hesitation about cutting them out.

There is enough evidence available today to justify heeding the long-term consequences of uterine or ovarian removal. Even research articles warn that: "Rather than being simply a container for pregnancy and the vehicle for parturition (act of childbirth), the uterus must be regarded as an endocrine (hormone producing) organ with an important systemic (body-wide) effect. Likewise, the menstrual cycle needs to be viewed as more than a 'curse' or a nuisance which women must bear in order to maintain their reproductive ability. Rather, it becomes an important component of their cardiovascular advantage."[140]

In 1994, 93,000 women died from strokes, compared to 60,000 men.[141] What do hysterectomies really cost the American public?

6

Atherosclerosis:
Inevitable Artery Plaque Build-Up

The mystery of how premenopausal hysterectomies lead to a 3-fold increase in cardiovascular disease continues to be revealed in this chapter.[142]

Cardiovascular disease results from both:

1.   High blood pressure (chapter 5) and
2.   **Atherosclerosis** (fat build up on artery walls).

Atherosclerosis. I knew the word, but had not paid much attention to it. I watched my diet and felt I did not have to worry about it until I at least reached my grandmother's age. Before I conducted the research for this book, I naively believed that high blood pressure was the only increased risk for coronary heart disease resulting from my hysterectomy. After the surgery, when laboratory tests showed high cholesterol, I did not associate it with the operation. With my experience as a laboratory medical technologist, I knew labs can make errors. So, never having had high cholesterol before, I didn't believe the report could be correct.

However, I began uncovering numerous articles, all of which reached the same disturbing conclusion. Articles with titles such as *The Degree of Coronary Atherosclerosis in Bilaterally Oophorectomized (both ovaries removed) Women,* leave little doubt that there is a connection between loss of ovaries, or ovarian function, and atherosclerosis.[143] When my search kept turning up many studies published worldwide, all indicating a direct connection of hysterectomies and oophorectomies to atherosclerosis, I realized I needed to know more about it.

To distinguish the difference between **atherosclerosis** and arteriosclerosis, they are defined as:

Atherosclerosis: changes to the inside lining of arteries by the accumulation of lipids (fats), complex carbohydrates, blood and blood products, fibrous tissue, and calcium deposits.[144] This accumulation is known as plaque.

Arteriosclerosis: degenerative changes in arteries which result in thickening of the walls, and loss of elasticity, and sometimes calcium deposits.[145]

Studies indicate that premenopausal women have a much lower incidence of cardiovascular disease than men, but after menopause, women's heart disease increases and eventually reaches the same rate as men.[146] The common theory is that before menopause, ovarian hormones provide protection from cardiovascular diseases.[147]

Medical literature indicates, however, that there is a debate going on as to whether natural menopause, by itself, increases the risk of a heart attack. Some researchers claim their statistical analysis reveals no important increase in the risk of coronary heart disease in postmenopausal women.[148] Others find when plotting deaths from heart disease against age, it is not menopause, but just aging alone that is responsible for the increased risk.[149]

Part of the reason for this worldwide debate is that investigators, themselves, state that the underlying mechanisms as to why premenopausal women have a lower risk of heart disease have not been clearly understood, triggering further research in this area.[150]

Early Menopause And
Increased Risk Of Cardiovascular Disease

Even though researchers disagree about whether there is an increased risk of heart disease with natural menopause, the literature shows there is an association between early decreased ovarian function and increased risk of atherosclerotic cardiovascular disease.[151] One way investigators have reached this conclusion is the finding, at autopsies, of increased fat deposits in the arteries of women who experienced early menopause and died from heart attacks.[152]

Early fat build-up is also found in oophorectomized women, as their arteries contain 10 to 45% more plaque, compared to women with ovaries at comparable ages.[153] Women and doctors do not connect this detrimental effect to ovarian removal, because of the length of time required for the excess plaque to show up. Studies looking into how long it takes, reveal that in 10 years there is significantly more severe coronary artery disease, with an average of 14.3 years for the excessive atherosclerosis to become apparent.[154]

Studies like these, on both early menopausal and oophorectomized women, keep confirming that early loss of ovarian function leads to an increased risk of atherosclerosis and coronary heart disease.[155] Yet, as discussed in chapter 3, early menopause is exactly what hysterectomies can create.[156] The tragedy is, the younger women are when they become menopausal, the more pronounced is their risk of cardiovascular disease and heart attacks, or strokes, because they are exposed to more years of decreased hormone production.[157]

This increased jeopardy becomes crucial due to the fact that in the United States 76.6% of hysterectomies, or 425,000 annually, are performed on women before they reach 50, the average age of menopause.[158] It becomes even more crucial when the numbers also reveal 12.8% (71,000 women) are under 30, and the average age of a woman undergoing surgery is only 42.7 years. With these large numbers of women subjected to potentially disrupted hormone balance, years earlier than normal menopause, it behooves all of us to take a look at how hysterectomies effect women's hearts.

1.   Estrogen's Beneficial Effects For The Heart

As long ago as 1953, studies were beginning to show evidence of a relationship between lack of estrogen and plaque build-up in the arteries of the heart.[159] When oophorectomized women take estrogen, studies show that their increased risk of heart disease normalizes to a no greater risk than that found in premenopausal women.[160] Estrogen use has also been shown to reduce women's death rate from 30.2 to 12.8 per 10,000.[161] These results can be understood when we look at the many functions estrogen performs which provide cardiovascular protection.

A.   Estrogen Alters Ratio Of Fats In The Blood

There is an overwhelming amount of evidence proving that estrogen influences the concentration of cholesterol and the types of lipoproteins (fats) in the blood. Part of the reason for this intimate involvement is that the ovaries utilize cholesterol to manufacture estrogen, progesterone, and testosterone, which in turn effect some of the major fats associated with cardiovascular health.[162] The ones that have been investigated the most intensely are *high-density-lipoproteins* (HDL), *low-density-lipoproteins*

(LDL), and *very-low-density-lipoproteins* (VLDL). These fats take part in transporting cholesterol through the body.[163] Researchers feel that their levels in the blood are measurable indicators of cardiovascular health.

1.   **High-density-lipoproteins (HDL)**

HDL is the smallest and most dense lipoprotein. It beneficially performs the role of pulling cholesterol out of the body by transporting it to the liver for removal.[164] This "cleaning up action" removes excess cholesterol, and helps to prevent clogged arteries. Therefore, having higher levels of HDL is desirable.

The role of ovarian estrogen in maintaining beneficial high levels has been clearly shown in numerous studies. Premenopausal women always have higher levels of HDL than men, and when women have their ovaries removed, their HDL levels drop 27% lower than those which are found in women who have not lost their ovaries.[165]

2.   **Low-density-lipoproteins (LDL) And Very-low-density-lipoproteins (VLDL)**

Premenopausal women not only have higher levels of HDL, as compared to post-menopausal women, they also have lower levels of LDL.[166] As estrogen decreases at menopause, LDL increases to levels that are closer to those naturally found in men.[167] Neither LDL, nor VLDL, performs the same type of cleaning up efficiency as HDL, and they are easily incorporated into plaque, which attaches to artery walls.[168] These simultaneous events are part of what contribute to hardening of the arteries, especially the arteries of the heart, resulting in an increased risk of coronary heart disease and heart attacks.

The ability of estrogen to lower LDL levels has also been clearly demonstrated. When oophorectomized and postmenopausal women are given oral estrogen, their LDL levels decrease along with a simultaneous increase in their HDL levels.[169]

HRT Provides Conflicting Results

There is a great deal of conflict in the literature regarding the outcomes of hormone replacement therapy. One of its goals is to restore women's HDL and LDL levels to that seen in premenopausal women. Many studies show a regimen of estrogen and progesterone provides the desired effect of increasing HDL and lowering LDL.[170] Others, however, indicate that progesterone may neutralize estrogen's ability to increase HDL, although the beneficial effects of lowered LDL levels are obtained.[171] Still others indicate that, while the addition of progesterone does not have an adverse effect, greater beneficial changes are seen in the women who received only estrogen.[172]

These differences in response may depend in part on the types of estrogens and progesterones used, as well as how many days of the month women take them.[173]

Route Of Absorption

The changes in HDL and LDL levels created by oral therapy are generally viewed to be beneficial for the prevention of cardiovascular disease.[174] However, oral estrogen's ability to raise HDL levels is due, in part, to what is termed the "first-pass" effect on the liver.[175] It is a result of the liver's response to the ingestion of estrogens which were not manufactured in the body itself. This effect is not seen with the more recently available hormone patches or creams. Since they are administered through the skin, the estrogen does not have to go through the digestive system first. This difference with skin absorption means that HDL levels do not rise to the same degree as that seen with oral routes, but the beneficial reduction in LDL does occur.[176]

The fact that skin absorption does not increase HDL levels may not diminish estrogen's cardiovascular benefits. Researchers analyzing the data have consistently concluded that the change in the HDL and LDL levels created by estrogen can only account for approximately 20-25% of the entire cardiovascular protection that is seen in women.[177] This observation is further confirmed by studies on monkeys. Estrogen-plus-progesterone treatment results in a decreased amount of fat build-up in their arteries even though there was no accompanying change in HDL, and their LDL levels increased.[178]

Results like these have led to a search for other reasons why estrogens seem to convey such tremendous cardiovascular protection. Researchers cite several significant additional roles of estrogen, which have come to light, as being responsible for the majority of estrogen's and progesterone's beneficial effects. They are:

2.   Estrogen Directly Influences Artery Health

Coronary artery walls are lined with estrogen receptors which respond directly to estrogen.[179] When the estrogen molecule attaches to these receptors, it appears to exert several beneficial effects on the inside lining of the blood vessels.

A.   Estrogen Prevents Plaque Build-up

Autopsies on premenopausal women show that the presence of estrogen receptors corresponds to an absence of atherosclerotic plaque.[180] This research, as well as other types of studies, demonstrate that estrogen prevents the plaque build-up that leads to atherosclerosis by directly inhibiting fat and other plaque-forming particles (calcium, fibrin, etc.) from adhering to the artery wall.[181]

1.   Estrogen's Antioxidant Action

When LDL undergo what is termed "oxidation" inside the arteries, they easily adhere to artery walls where they contribute to plaque build-up. Estrogen (17β-estradiol) has an "antioxidant" action that prevents LDL oxidation.[182] This action of estrogen is so significant, one study concluded that the accumulation of LDL on the inside of arteries may be an important mechanism by which either natural or surgical menopause increases atherosclerosis.[183]

2.   Estrogen Inhibits Blood Clotting Factors

Fibrinogen is one of the primary proteins necessary for the formation of blood clots in the body.[184] Its level in the blood is recognized as an independent risk factor for coronary heart disease, because increases are associated with the plaque build-up that leads to atherosclerosis.[185] Studies demonstrate that postmenopausal women who do not take HRT, and women with irregular menstrual cycles (indicative of impaired ovarian function), have both increased fibrinogen levels, and increased atherosclerosis.[186]

3.   Estrogen Inhibits Cell Growth Of Artery Walls

As plaque builds-up inside the arteries, there is an accompanying increase in the actual number of smooth muscle cells. When this increase in the thickness of artery linings is coupled with plaque build-up, the inside diameter of the vessels narrows even more and can precipitate a heart attack. Estrogen counteracts this by directly inhibiting the increase in the numbers of the smooth muscle cells accumulating inside the arteries.[187]

B.   Estrogen Acts As A Vasodilator (Relaxing And Opening Arteries)

A healthy flow of blood through the heart is maintained, not only by keeping the build-up of plaque to a minimum, but also by having fully expanded arteries. **17β-estradiol**, the primary form of estrogen found in **premenopausal** women, accomplishes this beneficial action by directly dilating arteries.[188] This blood vessel opening effect is not seen with **estrone**, another major form of estrogen, which is found primarily in **postmenopausal** women.[189] This appears to be another reason why women often lose their cardiovascular advantage after menopause.

When women orally ingest estrogen, most of it becomes converted into estrone.[190] As such, it does not provide the vasodilation which is beneficial for the heart's blood supply. This difference in the action of the various forms of estrogen highlights the importance of which route women choose for taking their hormones (to be discussed in Chapter 14).

3.   Estrogen Does Not Function Alone

A.   Progesterone

Amazingly, hormones affect the ratio of cholesterol and phospholipids in the red blood cell's membrane. When women are given both estrogen and progestogen (a progesterone-like compound), more phospholipids are incorporated into the red cell membrane.[191] As a result, the cells actually become more pliable, and the fluid surrounding the red cell becomes a more watery environment, enabling blood to flow more freely through the blood vessels.[192] This benefit of progestogen led the researchers investigating this incredible phenomenon to conclude that the addition of progestogen to a woman's hormone replacement therapy program could be beneficial to the cardiovascular system.[193] This theory is proven by other investigators findings that whether women receive estrogen alone, or in combination with progesterone, they experience an associated decreased risk of heart attack.[194]

B.   Testosterone

Testosterone, a major androgen produced by the

ovaries, may also play a role in protecting women's hearts. Investigators, reviewing the few studies that have been performed in this area, state they reveal that androgen deficiency is associated with an increased incidence of cardiovascular disease. In attempts to understand why, one area being investigated is its potential influence on fibrinogen and other clotting factors.[195] To date, there is not enough data available to make a determination as to its role. However, the literature states there is sufficient evidence to justify the initiation of studies looking into its possible benefit for women.[196]

Ovariectomized Research Animals

While conducting my research, one of the things that absolutely astounded me was the fact that the direct correlation between loss of ovarian function and atherosclerosis has been so well established, researchers ovariectomize animals (remove ovaries) when they want to study plaque or fat build-up in the arteries.[197] To determine which ovarian hormones are responsible for protecting against plaque formation, they give the animals varying combinations of the hormones removed by the surgery. At the end of the study, the animals are sacrificed so that the amount of fat adhering to their artery walls can be examined and measured. They use this technique because, without ovaries, fat builds up in the arteries so fast, in as short a time as 4 weeks, they can dissect the animals to obtain their answers. If animal arteries undergo detrimental change that quickly, human arteries must change just as rapidly.

When comparing 4 groups given no hormones, estrogen, progesterone, or estrogen-plus-progesterone; the combination of estrogen-plus-progesterone results in the ovariectomized animals

having significantly fewer fatty streaks in their arteries. Lower
VLDL+LDL/HDL ratios, which are indicative of decreased
cardiovascular risk, were also found with either the combined
hormone treatment, or just estrogen alone.[198]

The Net Effect Of Ovarian Hormones:
Decreased Risk Of Heart Disease

Overall, a review of the literature shows conflicting results
as to the use of estrogen and the risk of heart attacks. Some
researchers find no statistical change, concluding they could
neither confirm nor refute the hypothesis that hormone use
prevents heart attacks in postmenopausal women.[199] However,
many others prove there is a substantial reduction in risk of heart
attacks and cardiovascular disease.[200] Part of the reason for the
conflicting results is due to the many different hormone types
and routes of administration that are available. This creates a
tremendous number of ways they can be combined, each with
their own variable effects.

When looking at the studies as a whole, it is hard to deny
that estrogen provides tremendous benefits for women's hearts.
A 1992 statistical compilation of 35 separate studies that were
completed between 1976 and 1991, found estrogen reduces the
risk of coronary heart disease by approximately 35%.[201] One large
study, which included one-sixth of Sweden's female population,
found the women taking estrogen, or estrogen-plus-progesterone,
had a 25 to 50% reduced risk of a first heart attack, compared to
non-users.[202]

These statistics prove that starting on the day of surgery,
when this hormone is removed years earlier than natural
menopause, all oophorectomized, and some hysterectomized
women, are catapulted into the same high risk category as men.

Loss of the incredible array of estrogen's benefits helps explain why they have more severe coronary artery disease, and greater risk of dying from heart attacks.[203] Yet, very few studies have been carried out that look into the consequences of the resultant hormone loss and the lifetime impact on women's bodies. A 1992 British article sums up the magnitude of this situation with: "The indications for HRT and the effects of different formulations on cardiovascular disease constitute one of the most pressing but complex issues in present-day medical practice. These questions can only be satisfactorily answered by the randomized controlled trials that should have been initiated several years ago and the feasibility of which is only now being investigated."[204]

Articles connecting hysterectomies to atherosclerosis have been published in medical journals since the 1950s. In 1981, one doctor concluded an article in the *American Journal of Obstetrics and Gynecology* with: "Pending further elucidation of the relationship between hysterectomy and cardiovascular disease, gynecologists should consider advising premenopausal women who are considering hysterectomy on the risks of coronary heart disease following the procedure."[205] Other researchers warn: "In any case, physicians in practice should recognize the potential of the uterus as a systemically active organ whose removal significantly increases subsequent risk of myocardial infarction (heart attack)."[206]

After reading the overwhelming evidence revealing the intricate role ovaries play in maintaining a healthy lipid (fat) content in the blood, I knew my high cholesterol lab reports were correct. It was hard to accept that surgery could lead to an increasing amount of fat building up in my arteries on a daily basis. The 1980 article, mentioned above, was published 5 years prior to my hysterectomy, yet my doctor never advised me that coronary heart disease was a possible outcome. Now, however, if I had been worried about the possibility of dying from a stroke due to my high blood pressure—I was beginning to realize that I also faced the increased risk of a heart attack due to clogged arteries.

All hysterectomized women, even those whose ovaries are preserved, need to protect their hearts by monitoring their cholesterol and LDL/HDL ratios. Heart disease IS American women's #1 killer, causing nearly 500,000 deaths every year.

7

Osteoporosis:
Accelerates When Ovarian Function Declines or Stops

What does osteoporosis really mean? What does early loss of hormones cost in the quality of women's lives? Michelle's story tells us what it means and what it costs, as she portrays what her typical days have been like since she broke her hip 10 years ago.

Michelle lost one of her ovaries when she was 23 due to an ovarian cyst. When she was 54, a bleeding fibroid tumor led to a hysterectomy and removal of her other ovary at the same time. Partial loss of her ovarian hormones early in life, combined with their complete loss at the age of 54, set the stage for a simple fall at home to create dramatic changes in Michelle's life.

Michelle's Story

"No, no, the light is too bright. Nurse, don't you realize how it hurts my eyes when you wake me like this in the middle of the night, and turn on the light over my bed to change my diaper. I know there are many others you have to tend to, but when you roll me over in your fast efficiency, I feel almost shoved into the railing of this narrow nursing home bed. Don't you understand I just got back to sleep from when you were in here only a few hours ago. At least this is the third and final time you will wake me up tonight. Now, I know I can sleep through until they bring my breakfast tray."

How many times have I been awakened during the 10 years I have been confined to a nursing home, since I fell in my own bedroom and broke my hip? Thousands of times. I was only 70 when the fracture occurred, and at the time I did not know I had osteoporosis. I did not realize that one little slip would lead to an ambulance ride, extensive surgery the next day to put an artificial hinge in my hip, 10 days of hospitalization on morphine; then 10 long years of pain and being unable to walk. They encourage me to walk, but I am afraid I will lose my balance and fall again; afraid of another broken hip or more broken bones. The pain is too much, as I have not been free of pain during the entire 10 years.

Now, my daily routine consists of receiving my breakfast tray, having my diaper changed, the therapist coming to help me walk, lunch (which is brought way too early after breakfast—I am never hungry at the time), watching television, reading the medical newsletters I subscribe to, having my diaper changed, a dinner tray, watching more television, and trying to get some sleep before the first diaper change in the middle of the night. They are really nice and good to me here, but I am totally dependent on their routine, not mine.

Thank goodness my federal insurance has paid over half of the $600,000 this nursing home has charged over the last 10 years. On top of that have been all the doctors' bills and extras, like wheelchairs and walkers.

I wish they would make a wheelchair that would fit MY body and MY needs. They are all either too tall, or too short. Nothing is comfortable. Writing is difficult, because it hurts too much to pull myself up to a position where my hand is on a table. The mattress is too hard for my painful hip, while the egg crate pad they put on top for softness slips all over the place, and in the morning both it, and I, are lodged sideways in the bed.

If I had one wish—I wish I could get out of here.

My one regret—having to sell my nice, custom-made home. It was so lovely, but I have no use for it anymore.

Every night I pray for the world—that there will be no catastrophic weather events, no wars, no crime, or poverty.

If I could give the world one message—I would tell people to take care of themselves, so they don't wind up like me.

Michelle's story is not unique. This description of what daily life is like with an osteoporotic broken hip could be any one of the 300,000 who break their hips every year, leading to the 60,000 who, like Michelle, need additional living assistance. Today, 22.4 million women in America suffer from low bone mass, placing them at increased risk of osteoporosis and breakage of their fragile bones.[207] The literature cites over and over again: "Osteoporosis is one of the most prevalent musculoskeletal disorders afflicting the elderly population today."[208] It is so much more prevalent than cancer, a woman's risk of developing a hip fracture is equal to her risk of developing all three cancers—breast, uterine, and ovarian combined.[209]

How does osteoporosis start? Why does it start? Why do some women get it, and others don't? Why don't we hear more stories about our grandmothers and great-grandmothers breaking fragile bones? Osteoporosis was the last thing on my mind when I started the research that culminated in this book, but my investigation of estrogen immediately led me to the subject.

Bone is in a constant state of flux, breaking down and rebuilding every day.[210] Throughout the body there is an active ongoing exchange of the hormones, chemicals, and minerals needed to create strong, healthy bones.[211] It is an extremely complex interaction, involving a multitude of chemicals and hormones, all of which are essential. When something creates an imbalance in this process, the result is osteoporosis.

Two Types of Osteoporosis

It is theorized that there are 2 types of osteoporosis affecting different areas within the bones.[212]

Type 1, menopausal osteoporosis, is associated with decreased ovarian function, which, in turn, alters other hormones and chemicals involved in maintaining strong bones. When the body's naturally protective hormone production slows at menopause, or is compromised or removed by surgery, bone loss accelerates immediately. The resultant mineral loss creates what are known as crush type fractures to the vertebrae. The fractures start appearing 15-20 years after either natural, or surgical menopause, with women experiencing measurable height loss.[213]

In **type 2**, senile (old age) osteoporosis, disintegration of the bone is a slower process, some of which is the result of altered metabolism and decreased absorption of calcium. It leads to wedge type fractures of the vertebrae, creating what is commonly known as a dowager's hump.[214]

Risk Factors Leading To Osteoporosis

When looking at risk factors for developing osteoporosis, they are broken down into 3 separate categories: Major, Moderate-to-Major, and Average-to-Moderate. Only 4 risk factors are classified as Major. They are:

1. Menopause before age 45
2. Taking corticoid-steroids for 1 year or more
3. Absence of menstrual cycle for more than 1 year, excluding menopause
4. Personal or family history of a fragility fracture

Source: Reprinted with permission, Galsworthy TD. The mechanism of an osteoporosis center. *Orthopedic Clin North Amer.* 1990 Jan. 21(1):163-9. Updated per author fax (1998 Mar 11).

The absence of menstrual cycle for more than one year classifies oophorectomies as a major risk, and clearly shows the detrimental effect created by ovarian removal. Since removal of the uterus forces many women into menopause before the age of 45 (see chapter 3), it also illustrates the destructive potential of hysterectomies.

When women are allowed to go through natural menopause, around the average age of 50, they only fall into the 'Moderate-to-Major' category of developing osteoporosis.[215] Even though these women are in a lower risk category, they can still lose up to 20% of their bone mass in the first 5 to 7 years following menopause.[216]

The Chemicals Involved In Bone Maintenance

Hormones arising from the ovaries or testicles are critical to the maintenance of strong bones.[217] Some of the major players required for bone maintenance are:

Hormone/Chemical	Function
1. Estrogen:	Prevents the break down of bone
2. Progesterone:	Essential for building bone
3. Testosterone:	Needed for building bone
4. Prostaglandins:	Essential for building bone
5. Calcium:	Essential for building bone
6. Calcitonin:	Prevents the break down of bone

1. Estrogen

The importance of ovarian hormones is clearly demonstrated by CT scan's of oophorectomized women's vertebrae. They show that, as a group, they have statistically significant mineral loss in as little as 6 months after surgery. The loss continues to increase, becoming highly significant within 1 year of ovarian removal.[218] This accelerated bone mineral loss is confirmed by the findings that oophorectomized women, without estrogen replacement, are at high risk of hip fractures.[219]

The increased mineral loss oophorectomized women experience can be explained by the fact that the cells which build new bone (osteoblasts) have estrogen receptors, indicating that estrogen plays an active role in bone metabolism.[220] Researchers even conclude: "One of the most striking hormonal influences on bone in vivo (in the body) is that of estrogen, withdrawal of which results in substantial bone loss due to increased bone resorption (breakdown)."[221]

Studies reveal, whether estrogen therapy is initiated soon after menopause, oophorectomy, or even after established osteoporosis, the accelerated bone loss can be prevented and bone mineral density can be increased in some bones.[222] In fact one study found: "Thus, regardless of the type of menopause (natural or surgical), estrogen use appeared to protect against hip fracture."[223] Other research reveals: "Estrogen replacement in postmenopausal women clearly reduces the loss of height to half that seen in untreated women, an effect which becomes most conspicuous after 65 years of age."[224]

2.   Progesterone

Progesterone receptors have been discovered on osteoblasts, indicating that this hormone also promotes bone formation.[225] Indeed, studies on postmenopausal women with fractures due to osteoporosis confirm this theory. In one year, the utilization of estrogen-plus-progesterone therapy created an increase in bone mass by more than 5%, and resulted in up to a 50% reduction in fractures of the vertebrae, when compared to groups receiving placebo only.[226] Following this group over an additional two year period revealed that they experienced an overall 12% increase in total bone mass.[227] This research helps prove others findings that progesterone plays an integral role in the rebuilding of bone, and that it is: ". . . found to be extraordinarily effective in reversing osteoporosis." [228]

3. Testosterone

The presence of androgen (testosterone) receptors on osteoblasts, as well as studies using testosterone replacement, indicates this hormone is also involved in both building healthy bones and preventing their loss.[229] Even when premenopausal women have normal estrogen and progesterone levels, if their testosterone levels are low, bone loss still occurs. One study found that low levels of testosterone can even predict future height loss, which helps to confirm that this hormone plays a key role in maintaining the structural integrity of the bones.[230]

Estrogen, Progesterone, And Testosterone

Results like these indicate that a combination of estrogen, progesterone, and testosterone therapy may be the most successful form of treatment for maintaining strong bones. The crucial role played by the ovaries is clearly revealed when researchers conclude: "Sex steroids (estrogen and androgens) are important for the maintenance of skeletal integrity before menopause, and for as long as 20-25 years afterwards."[231]

4. Prostaglandins

Here is another life-saving function of the same class of chemicals as those found in the uterus and cervix. Recent studies conclude that prostaglandins are potent regulators of bone formation and bone resorption (breakdown). Ovarian hormones are critical to their proper functioning since both estrogen and androgens can affect prostaglandin production.[232] Further studies are needed, however, because it is not known exactly how they all work together.

5.   **Calcium And The Complex Interactions**
        Involved In Maintaining Strong Bones

When bones start disintegrating, the resultant calcium released in the bloodstream starts shutting down the parathyroid's production of parathyroid hormone. This hormone influences the ability of the gastrointestinal tract to absorb calcium from the food we eat. As the parathyroid hormone levels drop, the ability to absorb calcium decreases. Thus, a vicious cycle of bone loss is created, leading to decreased parathyroid hormone, resulting in less ability to absorb the essential calcium that is needed to rebuild the disintegrating bones. This can be pictured as a domino effect in the following table:[233]

Bone disintegration due to a lack of estrogen
  leads to
    increased calcium in the blood
      leads to
        decreased parathyroid hormone
          leads to
            decreased ability to absorb calcium
              leads to
                the body using bones as a calcium source
                (causing bone disintegration)
                  recycling back to
                    increased calcium in the blood

This domino effect helps explains why researchers have difficulty designing studies that isolate just one of these factors. Hysterectomies, by altering a few of the body's hormones, create a chain reaction that ends up altering all of them.

6.   Calcitonin

Another thyroid hormone, calcitonin, plays an essential role in bone metabolism, by inhibiting bone resorption (breakdown). Its secretion is also influenced by the amount of calcium in the blood.[234] Studies show postmenopausal calcitonin deficiency is reversed by estrogen therapy, demonstrating the important role estrogen plays in regulating this bone-preserving hormone.[235]

Reflecting great controversy, numerous articles appear in medical journals discussing the thyroid's intricate involvement in bone metabolism. Is it lack of estrogen, or the disruption of thyroid function, or both, that accelerates the disintegration of women's bones following surgery? Again, no one knows for sure how they all interact.

This is only a brief overview of some of the hormones, chemicals, and minerals involved in maintaining strong bones. The complexity and individuality of all processes in the body are demonstrated by studies which show that women with fractures from Type I osteoporosis can have estrogen levels similar to, or even greater than those who do not develop osteoporosis.[236] They also reveal osteoporosis occurs in only 10 to 20% of postmenopausal women, and not all women develop low bone mineral density following oophorectomy.[237] Today's research has not uncovered what other factors come into play, therefore, women cannot know beforehand if they will develop osteoporosis when their ovarian function is lost.

Many new chemicals are being identified and assigned

their letters and numbers as investigators attempt to determine their role in the bone recycling process. Reading the numerous research articles about them is like swimming through a bowl of alphabet soup. Isolating just one component at a time, it may take many lifetimes to carry out the studies necessary to understand the total effect the loss of ovarian function has on women's ability to maintain strong bones.

What is known: *Imbalance in the system leads to bone being destroyed faster than it can be replaced.* The end result: *Osteoporosis.*

Ovariectomized Research Animals

The real eye-opener came with my next discovery. How do researchers design studies to determine which hormones, chemicals, or minerals are most effective in slowing down bone loss, or lead to the building of new bone? Again, ovariectomized animals provide the quickest answers. Researchers cut the ovaries out of animals then, anywhere from 3 weeks on, they perform autopsies to see which group of animals has the least amount of bone loss.[238] In only 3 weeks, there is enough bone loss to determine which hormones or minerals have the greatest effect. Take a moment to read the titles of the articles in the notes for this chapter at the end of the book. Their titles alone prove the direct connection of ovarian removal to bone loss. The fact that this type of research can be performed at all shows how rapid the process of bone break-down and build-up is, on a daily basis, throughout our lives. It also clearly proves that removing ovaries accelerates this process.[239]

Why do doctors think human bodies work any differently than the animals upon which they conduct these experiments? If lab animals, without their ovaries, lose that much bone in 4 weeks, why can't doctors recognize that women, without their ovaries, lose bone just as rapidly.

One can respond, "Women are not rats, they are different." Then why do researchers perform their experiments on these animals at all? What good would it do to see if vitamin D or calcium helps save rats' bones, if human bones are not similar? There would be no point in conducting the experiment. The researchers themselves clarify this issue by stating: "In the present study, we employed ovariectomized rats as a simulation model of the postmenopausal state in which women are known to be a risk for osteoporosis."[240] The experiments on rats prove that oophorectomy, or hysterectomy which compromises ovarian function, creates accelerated bone loss, beginning the day of surgery.

Tooth Loss

Early in life, when I saw anyone without teeth, I knew I never wanted to lose mine. So I always made it a point to take excellent care of them. Now, as I went through the articles on osteoporosis, I realized that flossing religiously may not be enough to save them. I found a new concern staring me in the face: tooth loss. When looking at otherwise healthy postmenopausal women, studies conclude that body-wide bone loss contributes to tooth loss.[241] Investigations on ovariectomized rats, as well, reveal that long-term estrogen depletion contributes to oral bone loss.[242]

Sadly, this made sense—teeth are bone. Our precious mineral balance is just as crucial to our teeth as to our skeletal frame. As I read these articles, realization dawned on me that I and millions of other women are not only at risk of being a burden due to unhealable broken bones, but may be subjected to huge dental bills and the difficult consequences of losing our teeth. Again, the cure is worse than the disease.

Osteoporosis Statistics

Today, women represent 80% of the 28 million Americans suffering with osteoporosis or low bone mass, which results in 1.5 million fractures per year, including 300,000 broken hips. The cost of these breaks to the nation has skyrocketed to $13.8 billion annually. Fifty percent of hip fracture victims are unable to walk unassisted, with between 15-25% (36,000 to 60,000 women) still confined to nursing homes one year after their injury.[243] They become burdens to their families and burdens to the health plan providers. Since most fractures occur in the Medicare age group, those afflicted become an economic burden to society. Not only are their lives radically altered, but our whole society suffers economically.

This is just the beginning of the tragedy. Approximately 5-20% of those who break their hips have a greater risk of dying within 12 months, due to complications from surgery, or as the result of being confined to bed and unable to move around.[244] Yes, as many as 50,000 women die from hip fractures every year.[245] Their most common cause of death is pneumonia, followed by heart attacks, infections, and emboli (i.e., blood clots or other foreign matter in the blood).[246]

Why are the numbers of women with osteoporosis growing so fast? If the burgeoning numbers of osteoporosis victims were simply due to our living longer, then our life-expectancy should have changed just as dramatically. In reality, the difference in women's life expectancy between 1950 and 1995 is only 7.6 years (72 to 79.6).[247] There is, however, one major difference. In the 1950s there were not the millions of women hysterectomized, as there are today, for the 15 to 20 years it takes for the accelerated bone loss to show up as fractures. This long lead-time is why a proportion of our recent osteoporosis epidemic has not been correlated to the millions of hysterectomies that have been performed. When the osteoporotic breaks occur, the doctors' primary concern is how to help these women now with their broken and fragile bones. Like Michelle at the beginning of this chapter, the fact that they have been hysterectomized has become irrelevant, ancient history. However, the current research does prove that women who have had a hysterectomy, even with ovarian conservation, have significantly lower bone densities than those who have not had surgery.[248] Therefore, they are at greater risk of osteoporotic breaks.

A brochure distributed by a leading pharmaceutical manufacturer recommends that women who are in a high-risk category consult with their doctors about having bone-density tests performed.[249] All women without their ovaries, or who have compromised ovarian function, are in a high risk category. This cause-and-effect relationship is now so recognized, the 1997 Balanced Budget Act authorizes Medicare coverage of bone scans for estrogen-deficient women (i.e., women without ovaries).[250]

After a woman has a scan and receives her results, what are her options? What can she do to stop or reverse the process of osteoporosis? HRT trials do show that bone loss can be slowed and can even lead to an increase in some bones. However, HRT can never equal the intelligent efficiency by which the body provides the right hormones, at the right time, as they are needed, ensuring the preservation of this precious, essential, functional resource—our skeleton.

Today, drugs have been formulated which can also help slow the disintegration process, as well as result in a slight increase of bone, but like all medications they have side-effects. For one medication, these include abdominal or musculoskeletal pain, nausea, heartburn, or irritation of the esophagus. They advise that it be taken on an empty stomach, waiting at least one-half hour, or preferably one hour before the first food, beverage, or other medication can be taken. To minimize side-effects, the manufacturer urges people to remain in an upright position for at least one-half hour after taking it.[251] When prophylactic oophorectomy is recommended, women are not warned that they may have to face this ritual every morning for the rest of their lives just to avoid the horrors that osteoporotic fractures can bring. Additionally, even with these safeguards, the stomach problems created by this medication can be so severe that some women cannot stay on it. What then? Where do women turn in an effort to save their bones?

Prevention Is The Key

All the literature agrees that disintegrated bones are so difficult to treat: ". . . it can lead to a life-threatening condition such as a hip fracture, making prevention a key concept."[252] Stopping the mass oophorectomizing and hysterectomizing of women, thereby preserving their full production of hormones, is a critical step towards prevention. The following quotations highlight the importance of this step. "In fact, the acceleration of bone loss which follows oophorectomy is somewhat more distinct than that seen in women undergoing natural menopause." "Unfortunately, once bone loss occurs, it usually is permanent. Thus, osteoporosis management should clearly emphasize prevention for all individuals at risk."[253]

Every woman, oophorectomized, hysterectomized, and postmenopausal, should talk to her health care provider about what steps she needs to take now in order to preserve bone strength, allowing her to maintain independence. Yes, independence! With osteoporosis, bones break at the slightest wrong move. Even stepping off the curb to cross a street becomes a hazard in every osteoporotic woman's life. They know that wrenching their body the wrong way can break a hip, and when it does break, the healing process is a slow and arduous one.[254]

As I reviewed the staggering amount of literature showing the direct correlation of bone loss to the lack of hormones produced by women's ovaries, I became angry that our medical system allows women to be jeopardized in this way. I realized I would rather die than become a bedridden burden to society, and be in extreme pain for the rest of my life. When I read about the large numbers of women admitted to nursing homes, and the up to 50,000 who die every year from hip fractures, I felt their pain and the pain of their families and began to cry. How many were the result of a hysterectomy? Until studies looking into this critical area are initiated and completed, we will not know the full impact that hysterectomies have on our society. However, this direct cause-and-effect relationship is too strong to keep ignoring.

8

Weight?
Now a Life-Long Struggle

In interviews with hysterectomized women, one consistent story kept surfacing. They either gained weight they could not lose, or lost weight they could not gain back. When these women heard I was researching hysterectomy's impact on the body, they asked me to find out why their weight had become a constant battle. They also wanted to know what impact the surgery had on their thyroid, and if it could affect their blood sugar values. They were now taking thyroid medication, and being monitored for possible diabetes, problems they did not have prior to surgery.

Upon investigation, studies confirmed that between 14 and 28% of hysterectomized women report having a problem with either weight gain or loss.[255] One article concluded that hysterectomy, even with ovarian preservation, is associated with increased body mass index (weight gain).[256]

To begin to understand why women's weight is effected, we have to look at how hormones and chemicals interrelate in a delicately balanced biochemical system with many feedback mechanisms. For the body to operate effectively and maintain optimum health, all the biochemical players are necessary. Each is like a brick in the foundation of a house. Pull one out, and the integrity of the house starts to crumble. This is why decreased estrogen creates a domino effect, leading to disruption in many of the body's systems, generating new conditions which appear to be unrelated.

Ovariectomized Rats Gain Weight

Research studies consistently reveal that surgically altered women may no longer be in control of their body weight. Once again, ovariectomized laboratory animals tell the story of the body-wide effects created by the loss of ovarian function. What happens to these animals during the experiments? They gain weight! Numerous experiments on the ovariectomized rats that are used for studying bone loss or cardiovascular disease show this. Whether the animals are measured in as few as 19 days, or up to 1 year after their ovaries are removed, they gain about 13% more body weight than the non-ovariectomized control groups. In order to minimize this, researchers use very controlled and matched diets, yet the ovariectomized rats consistently gain more. This weight gain is the result of increased fat, not muscle. At the same time, they exhibit a loss of approximately 40 to 50% more bone volume, which also reveals there is an even greater fat increase in these animals.[257]

Surgically Disrupted Hormone Pathways

Right from the start, abdominal surgery creates changes in the body's hormonal function. Studies state: "It is well known that major stress, like a surgical procedure, results in a profound activation of the hypothalamo-pituitary-adrenal (HPA) axis and induces a marked elevation in both plasma ACTH (adrenocorticotropic hormone) and cortisol levels."[258] Both of these hormones have powerful effects on the body, as ACTH influences all adrenal hormones, while cortisol is the body's natural cortisone.

1.   Thyroid Disruption

Thyroid stimulating hormone (TSH) is a hormone secreted by the pituitary gland which controls the release of hormones from the thyroid gland. It is one of the hormones monitored to assess how the thyroid gland is functioning.

Estrogen is known to enhance the response of TSH.[259] By creating estrogen deprivation, hysterectomies could lead to a loss of this enhancement. Since a normal functioning thyroid is essential for maintaining optimal body weight, this may be one way hysterectomies disrupt the body's basic metabolism.

2.   Growth Hormone Disruption

Thyroid hormones are not the only ones affected by hysterectomies. Growth hormone (GH) is a primary hormone which influences the body's metabolism of carbohydrates (sugars and starches), fats, and proteins, affecting how food is processed and utilized by the body.[260] Decreased levels have such a profound effect on the body that GH deficiency is now formally recognized as a specific clinical syndrome. The symptoms are typified by decreased muscle mass, increased body fat (predominantly at intra-abdominal sites), decreased exercise capacity, osteopenia (less bone than normal), unhealthy fat ratios in the blood, and a diminished sense of well-being.[261] Its influence on the amount of fat in the body is proven by GH therapy which results in an increase in lean body mass, along with a reduction in body fat.[262]

GH alters more than the metabolism of fat. Its effect on the heart could be even more dramatic, because research also indicates GH has a positive influence on the cardiac muscle, as well as on its function.[263] These roles are proven by statistics which reveal that low levels of GH are identified with over a 2-fold increase in cardiovascular deaths.[264]

Since estrogen stimulates the secretion of GH from the pituitary, and increases the amount that it stores, hysterectomies also create disruption to this basic hormone.[265] Studies on postmenopausal women help confirm this because they show that women who receive estrogen therapy develop significantly higher GH levels.[266]

3.   Cortisol Disruption

As a result of the domino effect, decreased estrogen ultimately leads to changes in another critical player, cortisol. Changes in GH create changes in cortisol because they cycle opposite each other; as one rises, the other falls, and vice versa.[267]

Cortisol performs many functions in the body. It is a primary player in the body's metabolism, as revealed in the following table.

Table 6   **Cortisol's Role In The Body**[268]

Stimulates:	a) Protein breakdown, resulting in b) More amino acids absorbed or converted to glucose (sugar) in the liver
Inhibits cells from:	a) Absorbing and utilizing glucose (sugar), their source of energy

The multitude of functions that both cortisol and GH perform in the body are so far reaching and profound, it is difficult to assess the full impact and numerous changes hysterectomized women undergo when their levels are altered.

4.   Insulin And Glucose Disruption

Alterations in GH and cortisol help create changes in yet another player, insulin.[269] Insulin is not just the body's essential regulator of blood sugar levels, it is also important in protein and fat metabolism.[270] Primarily acting in the muscles, fat, and liver, it functions at the level of the ovary as well (although its physiological function in the ovary is still poorly understood).[271]

Healthy functioning of insulin is of paramount importance because our cells require sugar for energy.[272] When there is a sufficient amount of energy, the excess sugar is converted into glycogen. This glycogen is then stored in the muscles and liver, so it will be available when energy is needed in the future.

Insulin Resistance

Normally, when sugar (glucose) is ingested, insulin levels rise, allowing the cells to absorb the sugar. It is an extremely complex process which can be disrupted in many ways. Sometimes there will be enough insulin, but the cells still cannot absorb the sugar if insulin's action is impaired in any way. Even though the insulin is available, something is blocking its ability to function. The sugar then stays in the blood stream, with the cells unable to absorb the energy they need. This creates a problem within the body similar to insufficient insulin. Since the cells cannot absorb the sugar they need, the body responds by increasing its levels of insulin in an attempt to absorb the sugar the cells need. This condition is known as insulin resistance (IR).[273]

Glucose tolerance tests (GTT) are utilized to determine the body's insulin response. When GTT values fall in between a normal response and a full diabetic condition, it reflects what is termed "Impaired Glucose Tolerance," and indicates that the individual is developing insulin resistance. Investigators have identified that a subgroup of genetically predisposed individuals, who evolve into the non-insulin-dependent type of diabetes (known as NIDDM), begin with insulin resistance.[274]

Insulin resistance is important because it appears to be a central factor in cardiovascular disease. Many studies show this group has increased: arterial disease, susceptibility to atherosclerosis, and high blood pressure.[275]

Hormonal Influence

Researchers are investigating the complex interplay that appears to exist between sex hormones, body mass, insulin action, and the association of the menopause with significant changes in insulin metabolism.[276] Studies comparing women with premature ovarian failure (average age 31), and those who are naturally menopausal, against a control group with normal functioning ovaries, reveal that estrogen deprivation leads to a greater impact on insulin than aging itself.[277]

Ovariectomized rats also illustrate the connection, since studies show that loss of hormones effect the initial absorption of sugar, as well as the manufacturing of glycogen for storage in the muscles and the liver. After ovaries are removed, both estrogen and progesterone are required to restore normal sugar metabolism.[278]

Studies, which show that women on some forms of estrogen therapy experience a beneficial improvement in fasting insulin values, help confirm estrogen's importance in maintaining normal insulin sensitivity.[279] Its role is further proven by studies utilizing ovariectomized rats. After their ovaries are removed, they developed higher insulin levels. Upon treatment with either estrogen, or estrogen-plus-progesterone, normal values are restored.[280]

These crucial aspects of basic body metabolism have also been shown to be compromised in oophorectomized women. They exhibit significantly higher glucose and insulin levels in response to glucose tolerance testing (GTT), when compared with women who have not had surgery.[281]

Abdominal Fat

The sex hormones not only play a role in the metabolism of sugar, they are also involved with the amount of fat that is stored, as well as where the body stores it. Essentially, the more estrogen available for the body to use, the less total body fat, whereas more testosterone creates a greater amount of abdominal fat.[282] After menopause, even though the connection is indirect, the shift in the proportions of these hormones ultimately results in an increase in abdominal fat.[283] This shift in where body fat is stored becomes critical because studies reveal that intra-abdominal fat accumulation is a greater cardiovascular risk than obesity alone.[284]

Pulse Release Required For Optimum Performance

The hormones of the hypothalamus-pituitary-adrenal axis interact with the gonadal (sex) hormones causing spurts of hormones to release throughout the day and night. This is a crucial factor for the normal functioning of the body in everyday life. Disrupted pulse patterns are connected to many disorders, including jet lag, inability to sleep, and depression.[285]

Hysterectomized and postmenopausal women complain of both depression and inability to sleep. The secretion of GH in normal adults is tightly associated with the beginning of the sleep period.[286] Studies show estradiol levels directly affect, not only the levels of GH, but the frequency of its pulse release, proving that compromised ovarian function results in changes in the body's natural rhythmic hormone secretion.[287] This loss of the ovaries' ability to interact with these secretory pulses is critical not only for sleep and depression, but for many other functions throughout the body.[288]

Today's technology cannot artificially recreate how the ovaries interact with the hypothalamus, pituitary, and adrenal glands to secret their hormones in the extraordinary pulse pattern nature created, making this another important factor surgically altered women lose.

This is only a brief overview of the body's hormone interactions. They are incredibly more complicated than it appears at first glance. If you do not completely understand these processes, you are not alone. Researchers, themselves, are not exactly sure how all these hormones interact. What is known reduced estrogen leads to changes in the hormones involved in basic food metabolism. In addition, there is no way of knowing how many other systems in the body are affected by the inability to metabolize food properly.

As with every other aspect of the biochemical changes created in hysterectomized bodies, there appears to be a subset of the population that is affected. The deterioration in glucose metabolism seems to be influenced by the individual's potential to develop diabetes.[289] Why this happens is still not known. Researchers are conducting studies into this area because: "The cellular mechanism behind this insulin resistance and the role of low levels of female sex hormones as a risk factor for development of peripheral insulin resistance are not yet fully clarified." At present their findings have led them to conclude: "Thus, women with either low levels of female sex hormones or high levels of testosterone might be at considerable risk for the development of NIDDM."[290] A major indicator of this change is the development of insulin resistance.

The following illustrates the destructive domino effect created initially by decreased estrogen levels, leading eventually to insulin resistance.[291]

Reduced estrogen
  leads to
    decreased growth hormone
      leads to
        increased cortisol
          leads to
            increased destruction of protein
            and altered body metabolism
              leads to
                increased blood sugar
                  leads to
                    increased insulin
                      leads to
                        insulin resistance

Hysterectomies, by potentially creating this syndrome years earlier than natural menopause, leave predisposed women with many more years to develop into full diabetes compared to women who have not lost their ovarian function.

After seeing how a disrupted hormone balance alters the way the body metabolizes sugars, fats, and protein, it is no wonder why some hysterectomized women fight a constant battle with weight. In helping both oophorectomized and hysterectomized women, their altered biochemistry needs to be kept in mind. They not only need to be monitored closely for potential diabetes, it is also a disservice to let them believe their weight problems are all psychological.

9

Depression:
"I Can't Get Out of the House"

While driving through an unfamiliar suburb of Los Angeles, I constantly checked the map, keeping one eye on it, and the other on the unknown streets. The address I was seeking turned out to be a cute white house in a quiet neighborhood. As I rang the doorbell, I thought about why I was there.

Early that morning, a concerned friend had called about her friend, Sara, who had become too depressed to leave her house. My friend recalled what I had gone through, including my inability to get out of the house, during the three years following my surgery. She said, "Sara didn't have both of her ovaries removed like you, but she sure sounds like you did during those years when we were worried about you." Afraid that Sara might be contemplating suicide, she pleaded, "Would you go over and talk to her? Since you've been through it, maybe she'll listen to you." The anxiety in her voice made me cancel my workday. Remembering all the days and months when I frequently thought about ending the misery, I knew I had to try to help Sara in any way I could.

As I stood on her porch, I prayed for the healing words Sara needed to hear, because I understood the desperation she was feeling. I also knew it was almost impossible to think rationally without the proper hormone balance. I additionally realized, if someone had told me after my surgery that a hormone imbalance could be causing my depression, I might not have believed it. This knowledge, however, would have saved me years of living at the bottom of a black pit.

Answering the door, Sara kept the chain bolt fastened and only peered out through the crack. She was wearing a sloppy dark housecoat and her hair was a mess. After I introduced myself, she apologetically motioned for me to come in, asking me to forgive her for the way she looked. When I had called earlier to ask if I could come by, she thought the hour and a half it would take me to drive there would provide ample time to straighten up, both herself and her house; but found she just didn't have the energy. She looked relieved when I told her I understood, because until recently I had felt the same way myself.

As we sat down, my eyes were still attempting to counterbalance the sharp contrast between the beautiful sunlit day outside and the drape-closed darkness of her living room. I could feel myself going back to those terrible months and years when I found it excruciatingly difficult to accomplish anything around the house, much less get dressed, and almost impossible to go out and be around people.

I encouraged Sara to talk about the surgery and what her life had been like since then. Sobbing hopelessly, she reiterated that five months previously she had her uterus and one ovary removed. The doctor saved her other ovary because she was only 35 years old. He did not prescribe any hormones, assuring her that she would not need them because one ovary produced enough. The medical diagnosis which led to the surgery was endometriosis (lining of uterus found in abnormal locations) and an ovarian cyst. She had been suffering from endometriosis for years, so when the ovarian cyst developed, the doctor suggested that surgery could take care of both of them at the same time. At this suggestion, she figured why not let the doctor remove what has been so troublesome? She had no children and didn't expect to have any in the future. The doctor assured her that after a 6 week medical leave, she would go back to work feeling better than ever, no longer having to deal with the endometriosis.

The 6 weeks passed uneventfully. She went to work during the seventh week, but felt she had to drag herself through each day. Brushing it off, she reasoned that after major surgery it would take some time for her energy to spring back. Over the next several weeks, however, she found it increasingly difficult to get up and out the door in the morning. Rationalizing that maybe she wasn't ready for full time work, she started taking days off, but soon found that even three days a week was more than she could handle. Finally, not able to leave the house at all, she began staying home on disability. Not understanding what was happening to her, or how long this would last, she began to develop a great deal of fear over the possibility of losing her job. Since the surgery, she had returned to the doctor every few weeks, attempting to find out what was wrong. He kept insisting she shouldn't be feeling this way and that what she really needed was to see a psychiatrist. "How can I afford one, when I can't even work?" she asked me as her tear-filled eyes pleaded for an answer.

Having spent so many days in the same despair myself, my heart went out to her. I told her how it had taken the right combination of hormones to get me back on my feet. I explained that surgery could have made her remaining ovary shut down temporarily, or permanently, if its blood and nerve supplies were cut. Even though the doctor stated she should be getting enough estrogen, studies have proven that this shutdown can often occur.

Her symptoms were so similar to the ones I experienced as a result of hormone deprivation, it sounded as if this was what had happened to her.

We talked for several hours. However, nothing I said seemed to make any difference. Every time I suggested hormone therapy, she insisted her doctor must be right. "How can this all be from a lack of hormones, when my doctor says I still produce them?"

Sara had become a lost soul. Even though I desperately wanted to help her, I finally left, feeling helpless. On the drive home I made a further resolve to write this book, hoping it would be a way to help all women, like Sara. Women should not have their lives destroyed by the multitude of changes, known and unknown, which occur as a result of the hormonal disruptions created by hysterectomies.

Upon investigation, numerous studies reveal the percentage of women developing depression following a hysterectomy is found to be up to 26% greater than that experienced by the general population.[292] When the ovaries are also removed, the number of women affected appears to be closer to 50%.[293] Depression most commonly occurs between 2 weeks and 4 months after surgery, but can take as long as 1 to 3 years to develop. The consistent pattern of timing, as well as the similarities of complaints, has led researchers to recognize what has become coined as "Post-Hysterectomy Syndrome." The primary characteristics of Post-Hysterectomy Syndrome parallel what researchers find in surveys conducted within a year of surgery.[294]

They are:

> Depression
> Fatigue
> Headaches
> Hot flushes
> Sleep disturbances/insomnia
> Vertigo/dizziness
> Urinary symptoms and problems

Conflicting conclusions are provided by other studies which indicate that there is no increase in depression after hysterectomy.[295] These inconsistencies have led to an ongoing debate over the validity of this syndrome.

Addressing the wide discrepancy, two researchers stated: "Such clashing clinical viewpoints are best reconciled by extensive research. Unfortunately, however, long-term prospective studies of the effects of elective hysterectomy, using randomly assigned control groups and measuring psychological and social variables as well as physical and psychosomatic symptoms, do not appear to have been done."[296]

As long ago as 1963 researchers warned: "The psychological impact of hysterectomy must never be underestimated."[297] Yet, even 16 years later, others recognized there was still such a lack of information they were prompted to write: "A plea is made for more research in this area to determine whether hysterectomy is a factor in the etiology (cause) of depression in some women, and if so, which women are at risk."[298] Attempting to resolve these concerns, new studies were designed and implemented. Yet, today the studies continue to produce inconsistent results.

Why are there such discrepancies in the outcomes of these studies? There appears to be a multitude of reasons for the varied conclusions. The following are just a few of the difficulties researchers face when attempting to design studies to answer the question: Do hysterectomies lead to depression?

Experimental Constraints

1.   Surgical Variables

The tremendous number of surgical variables involved makes it is almost impossible to create studies comparing similar groups. These include: the reasons for the hysterectomy, the type performed, as well as the extent of surgery. As a result, many studies end up comparing apples and oranges.

2.   Physiological Variables

As previously discussed in Chapter 3, the uniqueness of the arteries supplying blood to the ovaries needs to be remembered and taken into consideration.[299] Some women's ovaries may no longer receive the full supply of blood they need to continue optimal functioning. This, alone, could be why the surgery affects some women, and not others.[300]

3.   Hormone Replacement Therapy

The studies do not always clearly report on whether the women are receiving HRT, and if so, what kind. This adds even more confusion and complexity due to the numerous brands of hormones available, and the multitude of combinations that are possible.

An example of this is reflected in one study that stated there was no increase in depression in oophorectomized women, when over half of them were receiving hormone therapy from implanted hormone pellets.[301] Since HRT should be alleviating their depression, valid conclusions cannot be made regarding the role of hysterectomies in depression, when some of the women in a study are on hormone therapy.

These are only a small percentage of the variables that make it almost impossible to design studies which would eliminate them all.

Commonalities

What needs to be considered are the number of symptoms a percentage of post-hysterectomized women have in common, among themselves, as well as with depressed patients. When compared to controls, depressed patients exhibit both increased cortisol excretion, and greater bone loss.[302] These conditions are often found in oophorectomized and hysterectomized women as a result of their decreased estrogen production.

Based on results like these, it behooves us to look for more common threads. When hysterectomy is compared with other life events that disrupt a woman's normal hormonal rhythm, a pattern emerges. No matter what the cause, decreases or changes in hormonal status produce similar symptoms.

Post-Hysterectomy Syndrome closely parallels the postpartum blues, with its symptoms of crying, irritability, and blue feeling that women experience after having a baby.[303] New mothers experience withdrawal from the high levels of estrogen and progesterone they produced during pregnancy, as well as a change in many other hormone levels.[304] Conflict exists as to which hormones lead to this depression. Nonetheless, again there appears to be a subset of women who are sensitive to these changes.[305]

Like every other area of research, investigations reveal no consistent answers. However, the menopausal complaints of depression and inability to sleep that some women experience as their estrogen levels decrease, closely parallel those of both the postpartum blues and Post-Hysterectomy Syndrome.[306] These commonalities, combined with today's research, provide the ultimate proof that the symptoms experienced by hysterectomized women can be the result of hormonal changes and imbalance.[307]

From my own experience, I did not know the medical explaination as to why my depression lifted after I started a regimen of hormones that my body could absorb. I only knew the days got brighter and brighter as the weeks went by. I didn't question how it worked. It was so wonderful to feel good again, I was just thankful something had finally made a difference. However, when my research uncovered many reasons for the deep depression, I became very excited. Here, at last, were biochemical explanations that made sense, clarifying why hysterectomies can throw women into a black pit of depression. Hopefully, with these answers, it may be possible to help the many hysterectomized women who are suffering with depression.

Biochemical Changes Created By Hysterectomies

Estrogen's Many Roles

Estrogen performs several crucial functions in the mood areas of the brain, and plays an active role in our feeling of well-being. Decreased levels of this hormone lead to reductions of both Beta-endorphins and serotonin, two important chemicals which affect our bodies in critical and complex ways.

1.   Reduced Beta-endorphins

Beta-endorphins are important chemicals which have become known as the "Beta-endorphin high" or "runner's high."[308] They affect our general feeling of well-being, as well as influence the amount of pain we perceive.[309]

Estrogen's role in maintaining beta-endorphin levels in the blood is demonstrated in studies of ovariectomized rats. There is a natural rhythmic daily rise and fall of endorphin levels, which these rats lose 5 weeks after surgical removal of their ovaries. When given a single injection of estrogen, the rats show a sharp single rise in beta-endorphin levels. When estrogen is supplied continuously, the daily rhythmic rise and fall of beta-endorphin levels is restored.[310]

Studies on oophorectomized women prove their Beta-endorphins are significantly reduced 6 months after their surgery.[311] Research on monkeys confirms this same drop after ovarian removal; however, it also reveals that the administration of both progesterone and estrogen are required for the beta-endorphins to be released into the blood again.[312] Progesterone's strong influence is demonstrated in studies on postmenopausal women which show that progesterone, by itself, can also restore endorphin activity.[313]

How it works is still not exactly understood, but this regulation of beta-endorphin levels leads researchers to believe that estrogen plays a major role in the functional organization of the brain.[314]

2.   Reduced Serotonin (5-HT)

Serotonin is a neurotransmitter of the central nervous system. Neurotransmitters are the essential substances nerves use to convey their messages to cells, enabling the body to respond accordingly.[315] Serotonin performs multiple functions in the body, including regulation of sleep, body temperature, blood pressure, learning, appetite, intestinal motility, pain perception, and sexual behavior, as well as reduces the breakdown of collagen.[316] In addition, serotonin plays such a key role in preventing depression and anxiety that increasing its level in the blood is the basis for a number of commonly used antidepressant drugs.[317] The most universally known is Prozac®.

Research reveals estrogen functions in many ways to assure that there is enough of this critical chemical available for the body. They are:

A.   Tryptophan Conversion

Serotonin is manufactured from the amino acid tryptophan.[318] Some researchers theorize tryptophan is only available for conversion into serotonin when it is in its "free form" in the blood stream and is not attached to its carrier, albumin.[319] When it is bound to albumin, it cannot be converted into serotonin. Both estrogen and tryptophan bind to the same sites on albumin.[320] When estrogen levels decrease, there are more vacant sites on albumin for tryptophan to bind to, leaving less "free form" tryptophan available for conversion into serotonin.[321] Ultimately, there is a reduction in the amount of serotonin for the body to utilize, which can lead to depression.

This type of action may also play a role in autoimmune diseases, such as rheumatoid arthritis.[322] Women experience remission of these types of diseases during pregnancy.[323] One of the reasons for this could be that the increased estrogen in their blood at this time displaces more tryptophan, resulting in an increase in serotonin levels.[324]

Many other hormones and chemicals are also being investigated, revealing that how or why this happens is not yet fully understood. Clearly though, however it works, products produced by the uterus and ovaries impact the body in critical ways.[325]

B.   MAO Inhibition

As if this wasn't enough evidence showing lack of estrogen can lead to depression, I was amazed to find that estrogen plays another role in maintaining high levels of serotonin, by acting like an MAO inhibitor.[326] MAO (monamine oxidase) is an enzyme that breaks down serotonin, once it is made.[327] MAO inhibition means preventing the enzyme from destroying serotonin. As a result, this second function of estrogen (that of not allowing serotonin to be destroyed) also helps maintain serotonin at higher levels in the body, thereby preventing depression.

This type of action represents another whole class of antidepressive drugs that have been utilized for years by psychiatrists. Two of these antidepressant's brand names are Nardil® and Parnate®.[328]

C.   Increases 5-HT$_{2A}$ Binding Sites In Brain[329]

Proof of estrogen's antidepressive role keeps piling up. Researchers have found that estrogen actually stimulates and increases the number of receptors for serotonin in the area of the brain known as 5-HT$_{2A}$. This critical area controls mood, mental state, cognition, emotion, and behavior. Investigators view this action as so significant in alleviating depression, they have labeled estrogen: "'nature's' psychoprotectant."

Within the normal population, serotonin levels can show a wide variation in range of activity in the brain, and the amount appears to be an inherited genetic trait. The levels of serotonin, as well as how it is metabolized by the body, are subject to individual variability.[330] The low end of the normal range is associated with people exhibiting suicidal behavior.[331] Researchers are theorizing that it is the women with inherited low levels of serotonin who become depressed when their estrogen levels decrease during menopause.[332] Women with naturally low serotonin levels could also be the ones who experience depression after hysterectomies and oophorectomies. These normal population variations may be another reason for the conflicting results in the studies that have been conducted so far on hysterectomies' role in depression.

Estrogen: Nature's Antidepressant

All these antidepressive actions of estrogen prove that the depression women experience after their hysterectomy has a biochemical basis. Studies performed on oophorectomized women confirm this. When tested for depression, before and after estrogen and/or testosterone therapy, all of the groups receiving hormones showed relief from their depression, a relief that was not seen in the placebo group (no hormones given). When hormone replacement stopped, re-testing showed a return of their depression.[333]

The connection between estrogen and depression is further proven in a study performed on hysterectomized, postmenopausal women who were "not complaining" of any symptoms. Even though they felt they were not depressed, after they were put on a course of estrogen therapy their psychological function scores improved.[334]

Such information clearly establishes a link between estrogen and depression. Yet, women who experience depression after a hysterectomy are turned over to psychiatrists who give them antidepressants. Today's antidepressants bring relief because they perform one of estrogen's many roles, that of increasing levels of serotonin in the body. However, estrogen may be what these women really need, as it not only increases serotonin by several routes, thereby alleviating depression, it also provides its additional health benefits for their hearts and bones.

When compared to those who have had other types of operations, or to the general population, 2 ½ to 3 times more hysterectomized women are referred to a psychiatrists—80% of them within 24 months after their hysterectomy.[335] Who knows how many women suffer in silence, like Sara, behind locked doors, no longer able to be functioning members of society. Without being told that they have a chemical imbalance, these women just flounder through life helplessly, attempting to keep their lives together, while in the throes of a debilitating depression caused by hormone deprivation.

Sara was single, so only her own life was in total chaos. However, many of these women are wives and mothers. It is not just their lives which are adversely affected, but those of their husbands and children. This surgically-created depression changes them so much, I have heard husbands or friends of families say, "When she came home from the hospital, she was changed." "She became impossible to live with." "She could no longer function as either a wife or mother." In one case a friend relayed, "After 5 years of dealing with his hysterectomized wife, the husband finally threw up his hands and left in total despair."

Over 100 years ago, there where those who recognized what is being proven by today's research into the brain's biochemistry. In an 1892 *Dictionary of Psychological Medicine,* one doctor, investigating the observation that a certain percentage of the women who were hysterectomized went insane, concluded: ". . . it is the deprivation of the uterus and ovaries and not the mere surgical operation that leads to insanity. The facts actually acquired strongly support this proposition." He stated further research is needed to confirm the validity of his argument that: "To unsex a woman is surely to maim or affect injuriously the integrity of her nervous system."[336] Another researcher, recognizing this more recently, concluded in 1978: "With the possibility of observing the effects of hysterectomy during this era, it has in fact been confirmed that psychiatric complications after hysterectomy, especially depression, are not infrequent."[337]

Recently, there has been acknowledgment that premenstrual syndrome (PMS) is the result of a change in the hormones which influence the brain's biochemistry.[338] The same recognition needs to be applied to the deep depression some women experience after a hysterectomy. All along, women have had their own natural, built-in antidepressant manufacturing plants. When hysterectomies compromise ovarian function, they disrupt this natural process, and women are left subjected to the possible jeopardy of having their lives turned upside down.

10

Fibromyalgia Syndrome:
How Can Muscle Pain Be Related?

Never having heard the term before, when a friend said she had fibromyalgia, I asked her to tell me about it. As she described her symptoms, I realized they were identical to what I had been experiencing—widespread muscle pain and the inability to get a restful night's sleep. These symptoms had plagued me for weeks at a time over the last several years. It had never occurred to me that this, too, could be related to my hysterectomy. As I interviewed more and more women who were also being treated for fibromyalgia, it became obvious that further research was needed to determine the possibility of a connection between this painful syndrome and hysterectomies.

Awareness of the syndrome is relatively new, only coming to prominent recognition since the mid-1980s. Today, fibromyalgia syndrome is becoming recognized as more prevalent than the much-heard-about chronic fatigue syndrome.[339] In addition, the possibility that they may be of similar origin is being explored.

Approximately 7 to 10 million Americans suffer from fibromyalgia, with women becoming afflicted 20 times more often than men.[340] No one knows its exact cause, but it is believed that surgeries, accidents, or trauma can precipitate the onset of symptoms.

Hormonal Influence

Upon investigating the cause of fibromyalgia, studies indicate that the hormones of the hypothalamus-pituitary-adrenal (HPA) glands appear to be involved, as altered levels and responses of these hormones are found in subgroups of fibromyalgia patients.[341] To determine whether the HPA axis hormones are affected by ovarian hormones, researchers checked HPA hormone levels in ovariectomized women throughout a 12 month period following their surgery. These women showed a drop in vasopressin, a hormone which originates from HPA axis. Since this drop was not seen in the hysterectomized women who did not have their ovaries removed, these results indicate that ovarian hormones directly influence the release of hormones from the glands of the HPA axis.[342] Consequently, surgery that compromises ovarian function may result in alterations of the HPA axis hormones, which could trigger the fibromyalgia syndrome.[343]

As a result, hysterectomies become very suspect, because several of the hormones which are influenced by estrogen appear to be altered in fibromyalgia sufferers. Some of the changes patients exhibit in the HPA axis hormones are briefly outlined below.

1.   Growth Hormone

Studies have found women with fibromyalgia also exhibit low growth hormone secretion. When these patients are put on growth hormone therapy, they experience a decrease in their pain, accompanied by an improved sense of well-being. There was no reduction in pain in the placebo only group. These results have led to the theory that a growth hormone deficiency, which is secondary to fibromyalgia, may be responsible for some of the symptoms patients experience.[344]

2.   Cortisol

Fibromyalgia patients exhibit further disruption in the HPA axis by demonstrating not only high levels of cortisol, but also a lack of its diurnal (daily) fluctuation, which is critically important for optimal functioning.[345] Disruption of cortisol is one of the hormones whose pattern is altered in shift workers, interfering with their sleep/wake cycle. This alteration could be one reason sleep is difficult for those afflicted with fibromyalgia.

3.   Serotonin

When compared to healthy control groups, patients with fibromyalgia have significantly reduced serotonin levels.[346] The role serotonin plays in pain perception is clearly demonstrated in fibromyalgia patients, as decreased serotonin levels are directly correlated to the intensity of their pain.[347]

Additionally, like cortisol, serotonin also plays a role in the second major complaint of fibromyalgia sufferers, the inability to sleep. When healthy subjects are feed a tryptophan depleted diet, creating a serotonin deficient state, they have significantly more waking periods and less deep (REM) sleep.[348]

The fact that low serotonin may contribute to fibromyalgia is strengthened by studies that show antidepressants, which increase serotonin levels, appear to be effective in relieving many of its symptoms.[349] This is further strengthened when the therapy found to provide the most relief is serotonin combined with MAO inhibitors, as together they maximize the body's serotonin.[350] Since estrogen performs both of the actions of these drugs, its replacement could be what hysterectomized fibromyalgia sufferers really need, rather than antidepressants.

With so many of the research reports stating that increased serotonin brought the most relief from these painful symptoms, and since estrogen appears to influence serotonin levels, I felt I needed to review my own estrogen use. If decreased estrogen leads to low levels of serotonin, could this be the source of the painful muscles I was intermittently experiencing?

For several years, I had been having trouble finding a satisfactory method to replace the hormone pellet implants I could no longer obtain. My doctor and I had finally settled on a natural estradiol cream, to be applied twice a day. I knew there were many days when I only remembered to apply the cream once a day. Upon reviewing my daily journal, I was amazed to discover that the excruciating early morning pain which awakened me so often, coincided with the days when my body was not getting enough estrogen. According to the diary, it took just two weeks of applying the cream only once a day for the muscle pain to recur.

Hormonal Interactions

Research is beginning to unravel and reveal the complex interactions between the HPA axis, the reproductive system hormones, and the immune system. Studies prove that the loss of ovarian function alters HPA axis hormones, and that fibromyalgia patients show similar disturbances in their HPA axis. As a result, researchers are theorizing that changes in the interactions between the HPA axis and the reproductive hormones may not only start the whole fibromyalgia syndrome, but could maintain it as well.[351] Since any trauma to the body has been known to trigger the onset, surgery, plus the added burden of hormone imbalance, makes oophorectomized and some hysterectomized women even more vulnerable to the development of this syndrome.

Hysterectomies are only one of the many possible events leading to the hormonal disruptions that can set the fibromyalgia syndrome in motion. Many young mothers seem to be plagued with this syndrome also. If one of the triggers of fibromyalgia is an imbalance of reproductive hormones, then modern birth control methods, such as tubal ligations, could become suspect, too. Studies verify that tubal sterilization can result in menstrual disturbances, which are indicative of hormone imbalance created by ovarian dysfunction.[352] This suggests that, with well over 350,000 performed each year, tubal ligations may be contributing to the rise in numbers of women afflicted with the disorder.[353]

This syndrome needs extensive researching, as thousands of women suffer painfully on a daily basis and have no idea where to turn for help. Not knowing, beforehand, which subset of women are susceptible to the development of this syndrome, becomes another reason why it is imperative to stop hysterectomizing women until more is known.

11

Bladder and Bowel Problems:
Increased Risk

This book would not be complete without calling attention to the increased numbers of women who have to deal with the disruptive, sometimes debilitating, and often painful symptoms of bladder and/or bowel dysfunction following gynecological surgery. Surgery involving either the rectum or uterus can result in damage to the nerve complex which supplies the area.[354] So, it is no surprise an examination of the literature reveals that a higher percentage of hysterectomized women show more symptoms related to both bladder and bowel problems, than women who have not undergone a hysterectomy. Several different types of dysfunction can occur.

1.   Urinary Incontinence

Like many of the conditions related to hysterectomy, there are two groups of women who are troubled by urinary incontinence. For the approximately 36% of women who experience symptoms prior to surgery, a total hysterectomy provides relief for 20% of these women.[355] While for others, these symptoms do not start until after their hysterectomies.[356]

In a study of approximately 8,000 women, they found that hysterectomized women had a 40% higher prevalence of daily urinary incontinence, when compared to women who had not had a hysterectomy. This clearly demonstrates that surgical disruption to the bladder area has an impact. In fact, this study identified hysterectomies, along with obesity, as having the highest <u>preventable</u> risk factor associated with this condition. The risk was so much greater these researchers concluded: "Our finding that hysterectomy may independently increase the prevalence of urinary incontinence 20-30 years later should encourage reevaluation of the indications for hysterectomy and further study of alternative treatments for benign conditions."[357]

In another study, researchers examined the nerves supplying the bladder, anal sphincter, and the clitoris, before and after performing a hysterectomy. Upon finding a large percentage of these women with altered nerve responses, they concluded: ". . . this operation (hysterectomy) has a significant and deleterious effect on the lower urinary tract."[358]

The possibility of hysterectomies creating stress incontinence in some patients is not just of concern to the patients who have to deal with this sometimes embarrassing problem everyday, it impacts everyone involved in health care costs, including taxpayers. The National Institutes of Health estimates that 10 million Americans suffer from urinary incontinence, at a cost of over $10 billion annually.[359]

2.   Interstitial Cystitis

Interstitial Cystitis (IC) occurs almost exclusively in women; producing symptoms similar to urinary infection, including urinary urgency, day and night frequency, and pain.[360] Since it is not the result of a bacterial infection, antibiotics do not help with these excruciating symptoms. IC is not easy to live with, as more than 60% of the patients report that they are unable to enjoy their usual activities.[361]

In studying potential risk factors associated with this

debilitating condition, it was found that 44% of the patients had a hysterectomy, again ranking hysterectomies as the highest associated risk factor of all.[362] In another study, 37% of the patients had a hysterectomy or ovarian surgery, with a total of 79% having had some type of previous abdominal surgery.[363]

Researchers still do not know the exact origin of IC, therefore treatment is difficult, and no cure is available. Since patients with interstitial cystitis are 100 times more likely to also have inflammatory bowel disease, studies are being conducted to determine if these two conditions originate from a common biochemical defect.[364] At present, researchers do not believe that hormones are the ultimate cause; however, due to the fact that IC occurs primarily in women, a hormonal role is among the several theories being investigated, again, making hysterectomies suspect.[365]

3.   Bowel Dysfunction

Over the years, medical literature has contained conflicting results about the possible role of hysterectomies in the development of bowel dysfunction. However, articles published in 1997 are now reaching the following conclusions:

> "In this study, the relationship between hysterectomy and changes in bowel function is very strong."[366]

> "Constipation, interrupted defecation and defecation disorders in general are unfortunately common findings after hysterectomy."[367]

These types of conclusions are based on results which indicate that a high percentage of hysterectomized women experience changes in their colorectal functioning.[368] In one study, 256 women had normal bowel function prior to their surgery, but after being hysterectomized for benign reasons, 111, or 43%, experienced considerable deterioration in their bowel habits.[369]

Again, they do not know the exact cause of this condition. The possibility of physical damage, as well as the role of hormones and prostaglandins, are hypothesized as probable causes of this incapacitating disorder.[370]

A.   Physical Damage

One symptom a percentage of women experience is chronic constipation, characterized by what is termed as "slow gut transit time." This can be so severe that some women may only be able to move their bowels once per week, while others are dependent on enemas to move them even once per month.[371] Looking into reasons why, one study concluded: "We found a highly significant association between persistently reduced bowel frequency and persistently increased urinary frequency after hysterectomy." The researchers of this study feel this supports the hypothesis that both conditions may have a common cause—namely, nerve damage.[372]

Investigating this possibility, another study examined 14 women, hysterectomized for benign reasons, who identified that their extreme difficulties with constipation began after their operation. Testing proved the severe constipation resulted from a dysfunction in the nerves to the rectal area. The article ended by stating that further studies are necessary to determine whether this incapacitating constipation is the result of the surgical techniques used, or due to the individuality of women's anatomic structure.[373]

B.   Hormones

Hormones are suspected because many patients with slow

gut transit constipation are found to have low estrogen levels; and constipation is relieved for many women during their menstrual periods, indicating some type of hormonal involvement.[374]

Studies also reveal 34% of women report irritable, or functional bowel disorder symptoms occur at the time of their periods.[375] Additionally, a higher proportion of the women who have irritable bowel syndrome state their symptoms are more extreme during their menstrual periods, compared to women without chronic bowel symptoms.[376]

The theory of a hormone connection is strengthened by the fact that estrogen and progesterone receptors have been shown to be present in the smooth muscle of the entire gastrointestinal tract.[377] This indicates some type of hormonal action at this level, the loss of which could result in functional bowel disorders.

C.   Prostaglandins

Researchers have been investigating the possibility that some of the prostaglandins that are found in the uterus also play a role in bowel dysfunction. Increased prostaglandins levels are detected in a percentage of women who experience difficult and painful periods. When these women are compared to a control group of women without painful menses, 61% are diagnosed with functional bowel disorder, versus only 20% in the control group.[378] Other investigators have found that estrogens and progesterones affect both the manufacturing, and the inactivating of prostaglandins.[379]

If any of the above theories are correct, loss of the uterus and/or loss of ovarian function could play primary roles in the development of the chronic constipation which can follow a hysterectomy. Other possible mechanisms are also being investigated, but due to the complexity of the body the answers still remain elusive.

4.   Fecal Incontinence

Another disturbing disorder, fecal incontinence, also points to a disruption of the nerve complex in the pelvic area. Studies looking at women with, either urinary incontinence, or pelvic organ prolapse, find that 32% have had a hysterectomy. When patients have either one of these two symptoms, combined with fecal incontinence, the percentage who have had a hysterectomy increases to 50%.[380] In another study of women with just fecal incontinence, 39% were hysterectomized, versus only 11% of the control group.[381]

5.   Irritable Bowel Syndrome

The symptoms of irritable bowel syndrome are diarrhea, altered bowel habit, abdominal pain, emotional disturbance, and stomach or intestinal gas that can result in abdominal distension (stretching).[382] Its cause also remains unclear. One area being investigated is the possibility of genetic predisposition. However, like IC, a high percentage (54%) have had either a hysterectomy or ovarian surgery, with a total of 65% having had some type of previous gynecologic surgery.[383]

As with other potential problems that can arise from hysterectomies, there appear to be two distinct groups; those who had symptoms prior to surgery, and those who developed them afterwards. One study found 22% had symptoms prior to surgery. Even though after surgery, 33% of these patients were symptom free, and 27% expressed their symptoms were improved, 20% had no change, and 20% experienced an increase in their symptoms. For women who had no problems initially, 9% developed irritable bowel syndrome after their hysterectomy.[384]

Other researchers question these results, stating that it may be the existence of irritable bowel syndrome creating chronic pelvic pain that predisposed them to a hysterectomy.[385] This problem is common enough to have still other researchers recommend a multidisciplinary approach which would screen women with chronic pelvic pain and then refer them to a urologist, gastroenterologist, or other specialist before recommending a hysterectomy. They believe that by testing patients for other potential causes of their pain, the rate of hysterectomies performed in an attempt to alleviate abdominal pain could be reduced.[386] In the United States, the percentage of hysterectomies performed for chronic pelvic pain is 12.2%, or approximately 68,000 annually.[387] Since 22% of the women undergoing a hysterectomy still do not find relief from pain, this approach could save thousands of women from unnecessary surgery, and from delays in obtaining other treatments that could help them.[388]

More Commonalities

It is important to look at the symptoms hysterectomized women frequently have in common—symptoms which many women state began after surgery. Over 50% of both interstitial cystitis and irritable bowel patients report being excessively fatigued and/or depressed, making hormone disruption suspect.[389] Studies also reveal that 42% of fibromyalgia patients suffer the symptoms associated with irritable bowel syndrome, compared to only 16% in the general population, leading researchers to conclude that there may be a common pathogenic mechanism for both conditions.[390] The common origin theory is further strengthened by the findings that irritable bowel syndrome and fibromyalgia are also found with a higher frequency of bladder dysfunction symptoms, all co-existing with a high percentage experiencing fatigue and depression.[391]

♥

This overview reveals that a high percentage of hysterectomized women have been identified with urinary and bowel symptoms, and points to the possibility that the operation may be a catalyst for the development of these conditions. Direct physical changes, such as nerve damage, may cause some of them. Others could be the result of alterations in the delicate balance of hormones or chemicals. So far, medical science has not unraveled why some women develop these conditions, and others do not. If there is a genetically susceptible subgroup, no genes have been identified with these syndromes yet. Therefore, women have no way of knowing, beforehand, if they are genetically predisposed to the potential consequences that surgery may aggravate; nor would they know if their individual anatomy makes them susceptible to damage of the nerve complex supplying their bladder and rectum.

Women deserve to know about these possibilities prior to surgery, since they may have to live with these types of outcomes for the rest of their lives. Again, the potential of developing any of these debilitating conditions is another gamble women take when electing hysterectomy as a treatment option.

12

Avoid Accidents:
The Body Never Heals the Same

If you take parts out of a car, will it run as well as before? No, it won't. Add to this, if the missing pieces are components of the frame, the car and its occupants become much more vulnerable to damage when hit by another car. Women who have been stripped of their integral parts become similarly vulnerable if they are involved in an accident.

Ten years after my surgery, my car was hit in a minor rear-end fender bender. The bumper was not too badly damaged, but I sustained a whiplash. I immediately began treatments which had great success with other patients, but my neck muscles refused to heal. After 8 months, whenever I was lying down I still could not lift my head, and had to pull it up with my hands. I would wake several times a night with numbness in one or both of my arms, unable to go back to sleep until the numb feeling left. This also occurred while I was on the phone. Since my job required a lot of phone work, and numbness made it almost impossible to write or hold the phone, I would be forced to stop working until it went away. Additionally, there were times when severe headaches made concentration difficult.

Since the damaged ligaments and muscles in my neck refused to heal, my doctor suggested that I see a doctor who specialized in a therapeutic ligament-strengthening technique. The procedure, consisting of a series of injections that strengthen the ligaments supporting the neck, has been utilized and proven to be very effective in helping people with my type of injury.[392]

As the treatments progressed, however, my lack of response to them prompted the doctor to ask, "How are your hormones?" I quickly responded, "Fine." At the time, 7 years of success with estrogen and testosterone pellet implants made me feel confident that my body was receiving adequate levels of hormones. The hormone level checks that were performed over the first several years of utilizing the pellet implantations had shown I was absorbing them, so I had no reason to believe they were not working well for me.

After several more months of injections my neck still showed no improvement, prompting the doctor to insist, "Get your hormone levels checked." Upon returning to the gynecologist who had originally inserted the hormone pellets, a small blister was found above the implant area. The blister had been there since the pellets were inserted 4 months previously, but I had thought it was scar tissue from the incision. However, upon opening the incision site, the doctor discovered that my body had rejected the pellets and formed an infected abscess around them. Unfortunately, the company producing the original hormone pellets that worked so well for me had stopped making them. So, my doctor had been forced to obtain pellets from another source. It was these new pellets, implanted shortly after my car accident, that my body was rejecting.

At last, here was the answer to why my neck showed no improvement. Since my body had not been able to absorb the hormones from the pellets, the lack of hormones was a major factor in my neck's inability to heal the entire time. The doctor compared all the treatment I had been receiving to "throwing seeds on cement and expecting them to grow." They can't.

Without the proper building blocks, ligaments and muscles cannot repair, either. Hormones are not only necessary for the maintenance of structural integrity of the body, they are just as essential for repair.

Once my hormones were re-established to normal levels, I began the injections again. For the first time since the car accident, my neck started improving. The arm numbness decreased to only one or two days a week, and once again I could lift my head without help.

As I looked back in my daily journal, the entries also showed a gradual decline in my reactions to the world. Without even being aware of it, I had started isolating myself from people. One big change was in the way I felt about bi-monthly meetings we have held in our home for years. On these nights, we open our home to guest speakers representing many different subjects. I loved the group of people who participated, and always enjoyed these evenings. On reflection, I remembered that I no longer felt like talking with our guests, and being amazed that I even had begun to wish we would stop sponsoring these evenings. At the time, I could not understand why I was responding this way because the group had been one of the joyful highlights of my life. Later, during my research, I found a study that corroborated this reaction. It showed that estrogen does have an effect on increasing one's ability to be around people.[393]

In addition, my journal entries often included the word "exhausted", and I saw that I had been having trouble getting through the day, much less going to work. Also, I had gained 5 pounds and did not understand why, since my eating habits had not changed.

It gradually dawned on me that these were the same symptoms I had experienced after my hysterectomy—difficulty going to work, gaining weight, and not wanting to be around people. Since I believed the pellets were maintaining normal hormone levels throughout the entire time, this experience proved again that these symptoms were the direct result of hormone deficiencies.

After the accident, had the doctors and I confirmed that my hormone levels were not sufficient, I could have taken steps to obtain the proper levels earlier, and my body would have had the tools it required for healing. Even though my neck was still not restored to normal, my medical bills exceeded $18,000. The accumulated cost was many times the normal claim for a similar impact, and the direct result of not healing as fast as women with a full hormone complement. After a few months of improvement had passed, the insurance company demanded that the doctor submit an estimated time and cost to bring my therapy to completion. He responded with what would have been usual and customary, had I been a whole functioning person. It turned out that both the quoted time and number of treatments were insufficient, and my neck still required significant therapy when the quoted completion date arrived. At the time of this writing, I still have not completely healed.

Ovarian Hormones And The Healing Process

Estrogen and Connective Tissue

Estrogen's importance to the structural integrity of the body is clearly demonstrated in postmenopausal women. Many of the symptoms they experience are caused by reduced estrogen levels, leading to a decrease of collagen in the connective tissues, resulting in an increase in their breakdown. These changes are so profound, one researcher concluded: "The evidence presented thus shows that postmenopausal oestrogen deficiency leads to a connective tissue disorder, with far-reaching consequences."[394] These disorders include osteoporosis, thinning of the skin, bruising, and urethral symptoms.[395]

Estrogen's effect on the collagen of the body is proven by studies which show women treated with estrogen experience a significant increase in skin thickness, when compared to those receiving placebo only.[396] Researchers have also found that estrogen, not testosterone, promotes the growth of connective tissue cells.[397] Since oophorectomized women are left in an estrogen deficient state, they face not only a degeneration of their body's connective tissues, but also experience the inability to repair tissues that are damaged in accidents.

Testosterone And Muscles

Testosterone belongs to a group of hormones that are classified as androgens. Testosterone and androgens are produced by the ovaries, testicles, and the adrenal glands. The testosterone secreted by the testicles and ovaries is much more potent than the other forms of androgens secreted by the adrenal glands.[398] So even though women still have adrenal androgens after losing their ovaries, these androgens do not function the same as the testosterone produced by the ovaries. In addition, as women go through menopause, their adrenal gland production decreases, making the ovaries' contribution of testosterone even more critical.[399]

The effects of testosterone and androgens are not confined to the reproductive system. They are also strong stimulators and primary catalysts in the manufacture of proteins in many organs of the body. Muscles are proteins, therefore decreased testosterone means a decreased ability to build and maintain muscle strength. Weak muscles ultimately put more stress on the ligaments and tendons which hold joints together.

Recently, numerous studies have been designed looking into the question of muscle rebuilding in men who lose all or part of their testicular testosterone due to illness, genetic defects, accidents, or aging. No matter who conducted the research, the same conclusion was found over and over: testosterone therapy increased fat-free muscle mass, as well as muscle strength.[400] When one these study groups was switched to placebo only (no testosterone), improvements in the muscles were not seen.[401]

If the less potent testosterone produced by the adrenal glands was sufficient to keep muscles healthy, the research studies would not show muscle loss resulting from loss of testicular function. If men lose muscle strength when their bodies are deprived of testicular testosterone, then it follows that women, who are stripped of their ovarian testosterone production, will also lose muscle mass and strength. Since women already do not make as much muscle as men, their ovarian testosterone production becomes even more critical for them to maintain strong muscles.

Again, I was astounded that testosterone, just like estrogen, performs multiple functions in the body. It is not only essential for muscle strength and repair, but also plays an important role in nerve health.[402] Critical to every life process, nerves are the vital life link for the whole body. Understanding this, as well as the many and varied roles testosterone and estrogen play in the structural integrity of the body, helps explain why their combined loss makes it difficult for oophorectomized women to heal.

Hysterectomies And Body Repair

The human body is a wondrous miracle that functions with its own feedback loops. Modern medicine's artificial replacement can't reproduce the body's amazing production lines that are so ingeniously orchestrated to supply more when necessary, and turn off or slow production when there is a sufficient amount. Oophorectomized and hysterectomized women, with either missing or compromised ovaries, no longer have this automatic supply line available. Even if standard hormone replacement works well when a woman's body is not stressed, after an injury these levels may not meet the increased demands required to perform the tissue repair necessary for healing.

Accidents that damage already weakened connecting fibers, combined with the inability to build strong muscles, leave bodies with little or no ability to heal themselves. Ignorance of the hormone imbalance created by hysterectomies or oophorectomies should not result in women suffering needlessly, or being cut off from medical care, when they do not show improvement with standard therapies that work for non-surgically compromised people.

This inability to heal without proper hormones has to be brought to light to both the medical community and insurance companies. Cutting out key players in women's delicate hormone symphony is akin to cutting wires out of a house's electrical circuit and expecting the rest of the house to stay alive and full of light. It can't, and neither can women's bodies when their ovaries and uterus are removed.

13

Sexual Enjoyment:
Where Did It Go?

My "asexual abyss" is what I call the three years I experienced after my hysterectomy, before I found a doctor who recognized that a lack of testosterone was the primary problem impairing my sex drive. When this doctor finally achieved the right combination of hormones my body could absorb, I experienced the incredible marvel of feeling good once more. After several weeks, I also noticed myself responding sexually again, and even welcoming the idea of having sex. It was fabulous to experience desire and feel my body respond. After 3 long years of feeling sexually dead, when I finally experienced an orgasm, I cried with joy. At last, I felt whole again.

However, I immediately recognized that there was a change in my orgasmic experience. At first I did not understand what it was. I felt a definite physical difference in the quality and strength of the orgasm, a difference so pronounced, I needed to find out why my experience had changed so drastically.

I found the answer in Master's and Johnson's *Human Sexual Response* written in 1966. They described how, during sexual excitement and orgasm, the uterus undergoes a 50% increase in size, which is combined with its movement and contractions. All are integral parts of a woman's sexual response cycle, and each contribute greatly to her orgasmic feeling.[403] Before the surgery, I had no concept of how my uterus was involved in my sexual satisfaction. It was only after surgery, with the loss of the feeling of its contracting, and the exquisite way the contraction blends into the whole orgasmic experience, that I realized how much of a contribution it makes. The absence of this sensation during sex was difficult to deal with. It is a loss of an entirety of feeling that cannot be replaced—like trying to enjoy a beautiful painting with a hole cut out of it. The painting is still beautiful to behold, but the hole creates a definite loss in the overall affect it has on the beholder.

This is not the only reduction in sexual response that hysterectomies create. Even though 8 to 12% of women state their sex life improved after surgery, I was astounded by the number of studies which show that an average of 30% of hysterectomized and/or oophorectomized women are not able to enjoy sex the same as before the operation.[404] Conflicting results like these show that when women opt for a hysterectomy they, again, gamble with the quality of their lives. The following table, listing the results from 5 studies, reveals the types, frequencies, and causes of new problems women can develop from this surgery.[405]

Surgery-Created Complaint	Cause
29% reduced sex drive	· Loss of testosterone
18% reduced genital sensation	· Lost sensitivity of cervix · Nerves and blood supply cut = loss of feeling and engorgement to area · Loss of uterine contractions
12-26% painful intercourse	· Estrogen deprived cells lose elasticity and thickness · Surgically-created structural changes
38% reduced lubrication	· Loss of cervical mucus · Estrogen deprivation

The studies identify that both hormonal and structural changes are responsible for these losses. When these changes occur overnight, the impact on a woman can be devastating. Even with this proof of how hysterectomies can interfere with a women's ability to enjoy sex, one post-hysterectomy survey shows that up to 70% of women complain that they were not informed of these potential effects prior to surgery.[406]

Hormonal Changes

Ovaries and testicles come from the same tissue when our bodies form. Even though testicles descend, their roots and nerves developed from the same area as women's ovaries.[407] The sex-organ-stimulating hormones secreted by the hypothalamus and pituitary glands, stimulate the production of testosterone in both the testicles and the ovaries.[408] Many studies prove that testosterone is what increases sex drive in both men and women.[409] One even concludes: ". . . our findings add further support to the accumulating evidence that testosterone but not estradiol (estrogen) is critical for the maintenance of sexual motivation in women."[410]

Oophorectomized women complain of a deteriorated sex life, expressing that they experience less pleasure from sex, an impaired sex drive, and decreased lubrication.[411] They also report diminished physical sensations in response to erotic images and physical stimulation, as well as absent or feeble (weak) orgasm.[412] Researchers themselves conclude: "Women who had undergone oophorectomy experienced a deteriorated sexual life compared to women with preserved ovaries."[413]

Another study finds when women undergo both a hysterectomy and oophorectomy, they report a waning of libido (sexual desire), compared with patients whose ovaries were preserved. If they are placed on estrogen replacement therapy in an attempt to correct their problems, they report little effect on libido, lubrication, or pleasure from intercourse, demonstrating that estrogen is not the answer.[414]

Testosterone by itself, however, may not be enough. Studies on women who are castrated, menopausal, or experiencing menstrual difficulties, all demonstrate the same results. They find that both testosterone and estrogen are necessary for the culmination of a vaginal orgasm. Additionally, women receiving both of these hormones report higher rates of sexual arousal, desire, ability to attain orgasm, and greater intensity of sexual gratification, when compared to those who received no hormone replacement, or just estrogen alone.[415]

Structural Changes

The loss of their sex drive hormone is not the only repercussion this operation has on women's abilities to enjoy sex. Loss of the uterus and its contractions during orgasm, alters the sensations and reactions that women are used to experiencing during sex.[416] In addition, removal of ligaments and other supporting structures around the uterus can lead to destruction of the blood vessels that engorge (fill with blood) during sex. Nerves can also be damaged, numbing the ability to respond within the genital region, furthering the loss of sensation. As with the ovaries, there is no way to tell which nerves or blood vessels will be cut and severed when the uterus is removed. The extent of this damage varies with each woman, which is why there is no guarantee a woman will come through the surgery, intact, with the same ability to enjoy sex.

Since women are not surveyed prior to surgery, it is difficult to determine how many are affected, and if they are, to what degree. It is possible that surgery interferes with a woman's sexual response to a much greater extent than the percentages show. Realizing the difficulties of predicting the sexual outcome in individual cases, one article concluded: "The negative effects on sexual life as a result of hysterectomy with simultaneous oophorectomy are important to bear in mind and should be discussed with the woman prior to surgery."[417] Others additionally warn that women and their physicians may jointly consider the possibility of sexual loss through hysterectomy or oophorectomy.[418]

The conclusion of one surgeon's article, which was designed to encourage other doctors to adopt his surgical closure technique, shows that this consequence of hysterectomy is well known. He stated: "This approach deserves careful consideration by the gynecologic surgeon who believes in preserving the sexual integrity of his or her patients. Those surgeons who use it will be rewarded with gaining other patients who have chosen him or her as surgeon for this reason."[419] Yet, even knowing all this, articles also reveal that: "Few studies on the impact of hysterectomy and oophorectomy on women's sexual life have been performed. This is remarkable considering the fact that the operation involves women's sexual organs."[420]

When a woman has her uterus from the beginning of her sexuality, it is impossible to separate out, or understand, the role it plays in sexual satisfaction. Only when it is missing, can she feel the difference. The loss is tremendous. Male doctors, who are mostly responsible for the current philosophy that female organs are no longer necessary after childbearing years, have never felt a woman's orgasm. How can they tell women their female organs perform only one function? They cannot possibly know the feeling of an orgasm, with a uterus and cervix, nor the difference in quality without them.

One woman's words about the loss of her cervix so closely matched my own experience, I realized that she and I were not alone. How many other women experience this same loss? She described: "The greatest change since the surgery is this. Before, each time the penis is pushed hard against the cervix, I would feel intense excitement deep inside me, huge waves of pleasure going from the area of the cervix all thorough my torso. This was by far the most exciting part of sex for me, the real climax. I've tried to be satisfied with the orgasms I get from stimulation of the clitoris, that is, mildly pleasurable contractions in the muscles in the front part of the vagina. Maybe I'll get used to it in time, but it isn't nearly as good, and I feel very sad."[421]

I knew I had to accept the way I now only partially functioned, but I was angry. Angry at myself for believing the doctor. Angry at the doctor for not understanding how women's finely tuned parts work together in such an orchestrated harmony. Angry that articles had been published well prior to my surgery describing exactly what I experienced. Why do doctors disregard these "side-effects", or treat them as if they were insignificant?

I found it even harder to accept the loss of my uterus and ovaries when I realized it was totally unnecessary. I lost my uterus because neither I, nor my doctor, knew that taking progesterone helps many women who experience heavy bleeding. I lost my ovaries due to the fact that I was over 40, and the prevailing myth that women do not need their ovaries past this age.

In addition, varicose veins wrapped around one of my ovaries caused the doctor to reason that the veins were responsible for my chronic pain. However, when doctors find varicose veins in a leg, they don't cut off the leg. So, why are ovaries considered so dispensable that they can be this blithely discarded.

If it were their own bodies, male doctors would not allow their testicles to be cut off, saying, "I don't need them anymore, I've had all the children I want. After all, there is a 1% chance of getting testicular cancer, therefore, I should have them removed out of fear of that 1% chance." Yet, testicular removal can be even further justified out of fear of developing prostate cancer, which is a much greater risk to men than ovarian cancer is for women. Removing the testicles, with its resulting loss of testosterone production, is one of the recommended treatments for prostate cancer.

Doctors don't take these drastic measures, though. They save men's testicles at all costs, because they know how devastating it is for men to lose their ability to have erections and enjoy orgasms. Would the doctors, who think that women's decreased sexual enjoyment is all in their heads, be willing to have the following surgeries performed on them?

Surgery For Men		Same As On Women		Result
Testicles cut off	=	Ovaries removed = (no testosterone)		No sex drive
Penis cut in half and resewn	=	Vagina cut and resewn	=	Loss of feeling and control
End of penis cut off	=	Cervix removal	=	Loss of pressure stimulation
Half of penis cut off	=	Loss of uterus	=	Loss of engorgement and orgasmic contraction

After having these procedures, would these men then accept being told that there was no reason why they couldn't enjoy sex the same as before? If they couldn't enjoy sex, would they accept their doctor saying, "It must all be in your head, and you really should see a psychiatrist?" I think not. They know testosterone is essential for their sex drive. They know that the contracting of the testicles and the penis plays a large part in their total orgasmic fulfillment. Why do they think that because a woman produces smaller amounts of testosterone, she doesn't need what she produces? Why do they think that the contraction of the uterus and pressure on the cervix during orgasm is any less necessary to a woman's fulfillment? The truth is that none of our parts, male or female, were designed to be so easily expendable.

As my anger subsided, I moved on to the next level of healing, having to accept that my body would never be the same. I had grieved for the loss of my organs 3 years before, but now I had to grieve over the loss of functions they performed—important functions—functions that I had not even been aware of, and had taken for granted. Since my uterus, cervix, and ovaries could not be put back, or artificially replaced, I realized I needed to accept that my sex life had been surgically altered, and nothing could be done about it.

Psychological Impact

In addition to the hormonal and structural ramifications created by a hysterectomy, the psychological impact of this invasion to the body should also be considered by every woman. My experience left me feeling as if I had been legally violated and raped. I did not understand why until I found research which confirmed that other women expressed the same feeling. In fact, it is so close to rape, when a rape victim talked about her pending hysterectomy, she was quoted as saying: "I know this sounds crazy, but it (having the hysterectomy) will feel like I'm being raped all over again."[422] Awareness of this reaction is recognized in the medical community. One world renowned journal article stated: "Women who awake from an anesthetic to find that, totally unprepared, they have lost womb, ovaries, or fallopian tubes, see what has happened to them as 'worse than rape' or as 'castration'."[423]

The reason for this is that a hysterectomy has many parallels with sexual abuse. These include violation of bodily boundaries, loss of control, disruption of sexual identity, society viewing a woman differently from the way she was viewed before her hysterectomy, and the vaginal pain afterwards. These parallels are so close, physicians are warned that, prior to performing surgery, they should attempt to determine if a woman was ever raped, because the surgery may bring back negative feelings that were dormant before the hysterectomy. The defenses of minimization, repression, or denial that a woman may have used in order to cope with past abuse can crumble during the crisis of her surgery, allowing the buried trauma of her prior sexual abuse to come flooding through, leaving the woman in severe psychological distress.[424]

In addition, it has been found that a high percentage of women who are in counseling as a result of experiencing physical and sexual abuse, as either a child or an adult, have a history of gynecological problems. This leads some researchers to believe there may be an association between violence and gynecological health, theorizing that these problems may have been created or manifested by the original abuse experience.[425] This is being recognized as such a cause-and-effect relationship, doctors are advised to include a violence history as part of their intake protocol for patients, especially when women report multiple past gynecological problems.[426]

Education And Informed Consent

Each person's sexual response is a very unique and complex process. There is no one thing that makes or breaks our ability to want sex, to enjoy sex, and to be sexually satisfied. Since there are a multitude of changes which happen to the body after hysterectomy surgery, the results of whether or not a woman can still enjoy sex may not be known until it is too late. If her ability to respond is destroyed, very little can be done by modern medical science to reverse the irreversible.

When being counseled as to the advisability of a hysterectomy, women everywhere should be forewarned and educated about how important the uterus is to them as a sexual being. The uterus should never be regarded as dispensable. Whenever possible, all attempts at salvaging the uterus, cervix, and ovaries should be made. As one study concluded: "The couple should be informed, for example, that some women do have lower sexual desire and arousal following oophorectomy. If this occurs, a vaginal lubricant, and a longer period of foreplay and stimulation may be needed. Women should also be forewarned that if they feel uterine contraction during orgasm, some change in quality of orgasm may occur post-hysterectomy."[427]

Both hysterectomized women and their mates can be helped when they understand her change in response, or inability to respond, is the result of the many physical and hormonal changes created by the surgery, not because her feelings for him have changed. Additionally, women deserve to know that the combined replacement of testosterone and estrogen can help them feel sexual again. Hopefully, this knowledge will prevent families and relationships from being torn apart.

Even with hormone replacement therapy restoring me to my original self, and as happy as I was to experience my new freedom from depression, the permanent physical change in my sexual experience was still devastating. Since none of these potential outcomes were discussed with me prior to surgery, I felt like a victim of our medical community's ignorance of how a woman's body functions. I felt raped of my body's ability to enjoy life to the fullest, as God had intended for us.

We cringe with horror over women in Africa being clitoridectomized (clitoris removed), to keep them from enjoying sex so they won't stray sexually from their men. Due to the fact that people are immigrating to America from countries practicing female circumcision and genital mutilation, laws have been passed making it a federal crime to perform these procedures on minors.[428] Television and radio shows which reveal that this practice may be taking place in the United States have shown people outraged and demanding that any perpetrators be found and stopped. But, what is the difference? There isn't any. The end result is the same—surgical castration can lead to the inability to enjoy sex. Yet, hysterectomies are protected in America under the name of "standard medical practice."

14

Hormone Replacement Therapy:
Critical to Know Information for All Women

One of the biggest dilemmas that all women face today is the decision about whether, or not, to take hormone replacement therapy. Making a fully informed decision regarding HRT becomes even more critical for oophorectomized, and some hysterectomized women, because they face a greater degeneration of their blood vessels and bones than naturally postmenopausal women.[429] The news is replete with conflicting information. Conflict exists among the doctors themselves, and arises out of the fact that the research studies show inconsistent results, confusing researchers and doctors, alike.

Ultimately, each woman needs to weigh the risks and benefits of HRT for her own individually unique body. In order to make the best choices, it is important to know as much as possible about HRT, the types available, and their vastly different effects on the body. The protection afforded, as well as the risks involved, vary tremendously depending on the forms of hormones used, their method of delivery, and their dosages.

The previous chapters have shown that women's bodies were not designed to function without ovarian hormones. Their loss impacts every system in the body. Since the degeneration is gradual, and many of the changes do not show up for 10, 20, or even 30 years after surgery, women are unaware of the slow, silent decline of their bodily systems. For some consequences it can be too late when they finally do surface, because they may threaten a woman's quality of life, and possibly life itself. To avoid such potentialities, oophorectomized women need artificial replacement of hormones. For women with decreased ovarian function, whether from menopause, hysterectomy, or oophorectomy, a vast majority of studies reach the same conclusion: ". . . estrogen therapy appears to be beneficial for menopausal women, as it probably reduces the risks for CAD (coronary artery disease) and osteoporosis, two of the major causes of mortality and morbidity among postmenopausal women."[430]

Unfortunately, fear of the much talked about potential of either endometrial or breast cancer stops some women from taking HRT. However, the actual risks of these cancers have not been put into the proper perspective—one that would provide women with the ability to make an informed choice. As mentioned in chapter 2, when looking at the risk to life alone, heart disease and osteoporosis result in over 500,000 deaths every year, whereas 43,000 die from breast cancer, and 6,000 from endometrial (uterine) cancer.[431] These statistics show that heart disease and osteoporosis, conditions from which hormone use provides protection, are far greater risks to a woman's life than the 2 types of cancers implicated to increase with HRT.

If fear of endometrial and breast cancer prevents some women from obtaining the benefits HRT can afford, then it is important to examine in depth the actual risks estrogen use may have in these cancers.

Risk Of Endometrial Cancer

First, only women who still have their uteruses need to be concerned about endometrial cancer. On balancing the possibility of an increased risk, one article concludes: "Although unopposed estrogen therapy (no progesterone added) increases risk for endometrial cancer, that cancer is relatively rare and is not fatal in the vast majority of cases associated with estrogen use."[432] One reason for this is estrogen use appears to be associated with less aggressive types of tumors, resulting in fewer deaths.[433] Also, the literature shows that if women take progesterone along with estrogen, the risk of this cancer reduces back down to that found in the general population.[434]

Risk Of Breast Cancer

A thorough search of the latest literature shows there is not enough evidence to make a clear determination about estrogen's possible role in breast cancer. Some studies indicate that taking estrogen may increase the risk, while others show no increased risk.[435] Still others indicate that estrogen may even have a possible protective effect, with a reduction in risk seen in women on long-term estrogen-progestin therapy.[436] Additionally, recent findings reveal that when breast cancers occur in women on estrogen therapy, as with endometrial cancers, they tend to be the less aggressive type of tumors, localized to the breast, and associated with a 16% reduction in the risk of their being fatal.[437]

Results become even more confusing for women who have a family history of breast cancer. Even though some researchers state their analysis of the available studies reveals these women have a higher risk associated with estrogen use; others conclude they find no evidence to support a differential in risk, when comparing women with a family history of breast cancer to those without a family history.[438]

The many conflicting results arising from these studies have led researchers to conclude: "Thus, despite the large number of studies conducted, we still need to know more about the details of hormones in the menopause in relation to breast cancer risk."[439]

"Definitive conclusions about the relation of menopausal estrogens to breast cancer cannot be drawn. The evidence is inconsistent, and if there is any increase in risk associated with use, it is likely to be small and to apply only to use of high-dose preparations (greater than 0.625 mg)."[440]

The standard dosage prescribed for estrogen therapy used to be double what is now considered beneficial levels for therapy. Some studies indicate it was the higher dosages that may have led to an increase in breast cancer risk for women who took estrogens before 1956.[441] Current research now concludes: "For the most part, the higher-dose preparations (greater than 0.625 mg) should not be necessary for clinical relief of menopausal symptoms, to favorably affect CAD (coronary artery disease) risk, or for prevention of osteoporosis."[442]

Each Woman Must Find Her Own Answers

Articles conclude that definitive answers on estrogen's role in breast cancer will not be available until the results from studies currently in progress, like the Women's Health Initiative, are completed, analyzed, and the findings published, possibly in the year 2005.[443] Until then, one team of researchers advised: ". . . a woman must learn as much as possible about the risks and benefits of postmenopausal hormone replacement therapy for her individual circumstances, so that she can make an informed decision about taking a drug for perhaps the rest of her life."[444] This is essential for women as researchers conclude: "In every analysis the lives saved from prevention of heart disease by estrogen alone outweigh the deaths incurred from breast cancer."[445] This chapter is devoted to providing a foundation of knowledge which women can continue to update as the answers from research studies become available in the next several years.

Finding The Right Route Of Therapy

The Forms Of Estrogen

Estrogen does not exist in a single form, nor is it produced only by the ovaries. The major form of estrogen made by the ovaries is called **estradiol**, whereas fat tissue cells manufacture what is termed **estrone**.[446] Before menopause, women have either more of the estradiol form, or close to equal concentrations of estradiol and estrone.[447] After menopause, the estrone concentrations of postmenopausal women become approximately five times greater than that of estradiol.[448] This is a result of the fact that the majority of estrogen is manufactured by the fat cells, rather than the ovaries being the primary site of synthesis.[449]

Since premenopausal women have less heart disease and osteoporosis, it appears estradiol is the form of estrogen which provides the most benefit for the body. Therefore, this menopausal shift to greater concentrations of estrone may be one way women lose their natural cardiovascular protection. As discussed in chapter 6, estradiol has the ability to dilate blood vessels, whereas estrone does not. This is just one major difference in the actions of these two forms of estrogen, and may be one way women's hearts are protected before menopause.

How much estradiol or estrone becomes available for the body to utilize varies greatly, depending on whether estrogen is taken orally or absorbed through the skin.[450] In addition, what kind of estrogens, as well as their dosages, lead to tremendous differences in the levels of estradiol and estrone attained in the blood, as well as their ratio to each other.[451] Even more importantly, no matter which route of therapy is used (oral, skin, or vaginal), not all women absorb hormones the same, resulting in further differences in the levels and ratios of these forms of estrogen.[452]

Understanding these differences is important when selecting the route and type of HRT to take. It is critical for every woman to find a safe route that will deliver the protective form of estrogen she needs, as well as one her body can absorb effectively.

Oral Routes

The vast majority of estrogen used in the United States has been oral conjugated estrogens, of which Premarin® is the most commonly recognized.[453] As a result, most of the information available today is based on studies of women who were taking conjugated estrogens.

After oral ingestion, a considerable portion of any estrogen is inactivated or rendered useless by the gut, and most of the remainder is converted into estrone.[454] It then undergoes the "first-pass" metabolism by the liver. In this process, the liver metabolizes it very differently than the estrogen produced by the human body.[455] Any remaining estradiol is further converted, creating a final product that is mostly estrone.[456] This digestive process produces ratios of estradiol to estrone which are closer to those found in postmenopausal women.[457]

Oral digestion of estrogen is so different for the body, researchers state: ". . . estrogen replacement therapy does not mimic natural or physiological hormone production that occurs during reproductive life and is, in fact, substitution rather than replacement therapy."[458] In other words, oral estrogens cannot replace what the body naturally provides. In addition, the liver is extremely sensitive to estrogenic compounds. This sensitivity can lead, although rarely, to the development of benign tumors (adenomas) of the liver. So far, however, they have only been connected to oral contraceptive use and can regress upon discontinuation of the contraceptive.[459] Even though these tumors are not cancerous, and not identified with postmenopausal estrogen use, the information published in the *Physician's Desk Reference* (PDR) includes the warning that they can be life-threatening.[460] As far as the potential of liver cancer, the manufacturer states: "At present there is no good evidence that women using estrogens in the menopause have an increased risk of such tumors, but there is no way yet to be sure they do not . . . . "[461]

While more time is needed to determine if there is a cause-and-effect of postmenopausal oral estrogen use and tumors in the liver, it is known they create changes in many of the actions carried out by the liver. The following table shows many of the altered liver functions and the potential problems that can arise from oral estrogens.

Table 8   **Functions Altered by Oral Estrogen**[462]

Function Altered	Detrimental Result
· Coagulation factors altered	· Thromboembolism (blood clots)
· Bile secretion is decreased:	· Gall-bladder disease
· Glucose metabolism is altered	· Insulin resistance · Reduced glucose tolerance (diabetes)
· Enzyme metabolism is altered	· Multiple effects · Jaundice
· Sex hormone binding globulin (SHBG) increased	· Decreased estrogen and testosterone available for body to use · Decreased bone mineralization
· Renin substrate increased	· Altered blood pressure

Function Altered	Beneficial Result
· Fat metabolism changes	· Increase in HDL · Decreased in LDL (less plaque build-up)

Even though oral estrogens cause the liver to produce what is believed to be cardio-protective levels and ratios of HDL and LDL, this table shows that many of the other changes created in the liver can be detrimental. Consequently, women need to look for alternative methods of hormone delivery, ones that do not go directly to the liver to be metabolized.

Non-oral Routes: Patches, Creams, And Pellets

So far, alternate delivery routes include skin patches, creams, and hormone impregnated pellets. Patches are placed on the abdomen or buttocks, allowing the skin to absorb the hormone over a period of several days. Creams also absorb through the skin and can be applied once or several times a day to an area where the skin is soft. The pellets are implanted into the fatty tissue of the buttocks or abdomen, where they are absorbed gradually over a three to six month period.

Non-oral therapies provide most of the same benefits as oral estrogens, plus they have several additional important advantages. These include:

1.   Liver Metabolism Not Altered

The altered liver functions described in Table 8 do not occur when estrogens are absorbed through the skin, indicating this route does not cause these detrimental effects either in the liver, or throughout the body.[463]

2.   Premenopausal Estrogen Ratios

By avoiding the "first-pass" effect on the liver, non-oral routes generate a greater concentration of estradiol than that of estrone, ultimately producing the more protective levels and ratios of estrogens found in premenopausal women.[464]

3.   Cardiovascular Protection

Since patches are a relatively new phenomenon, there are few studies available confirming whether they provide the same heart protection as oral estrogens. The extreme increase in HDL levels created by oral routes does not occur with the non-oral routes.[465] The rise in HDL has been considered one of the beneficial aspects of oral therapy, even though this is the result of the "first-pass" effect on the liver.

The differences in HDL response, combined with the fact that long-term studies on patches have not been completed, cause some doctors to hesitate recommending this route of therapy. However, when compared to either oral ingestion or placebos (no estrogen), non-oral estrogens maintain fat profiles more closely resembling premenopausal levels and ratios, which overall may physiologically be more beneficial for women.[466]

Furthermore, the rise in HDL is not the only role estrogen performs in protecting the heart. As discussed in chapter 6, researchers believe this can account for only 20 to 25% of estrogen's cardiovascular protection.[467] Non-oral routes appear to supply the additional 75-80% of estrogen's critical actions.

It could be that non-oral routes may even provide greater protection for the heart than oral routes. Since they are not involved in the "first pass" liver effect, non-oral routes do not lead to the deterioration of glucose tolerance testing, or higher insulin levels that can occur with oral routes.[468] As discussed in chapter 8, these are two signs indicative of insulin resistance, and are considered "risk factors" for cardiovascular disease.[469]

4.   Osteoporosis Prevention

Another major reason for taking HRT is for protection from osteoporosis. Studies reveal that patches not only stop the bone loss associated with menopause, but also have been shown to increase bone, as well as reduce fractures.[470] The fact that fractures are reduced is important because some medications may increase the amount of bone, but the bone produced can be weak and still fracture easily.

5.　　Relief From Menopausal Symptoms

Many women take HRT for relief from menopausal symptoms, the most noticeable being hot flushes, so bothersome for some, they can be their primary reason for taking hormones. Studies show that non-oral routes, such as vaginal creams, produce relief from hot flushes.[471]

Testosterone Replacement

Awareness of testosterone's essential role has been increasing, with some physicians beginning to include it in their replacement therapies. Pharmaceutical companies have also responded to the demand for combined hormone replacement by creating pills that contain both estrogen and testosterone. However, when taken orally, the same problem can occur with testosterone as with estrogen. It can damage the liver and prevent it from optimally performing its multitude of normal daily functions. This leads to the same side-effects that occur with oral estrogens which include nausea, altered liver enzymes, jaundice, hepatitis, and, again though rarely, can even cause tumors. Testosterone, as well as estrogen, administered this way may also result in electrolyte (salt) disturbances, causing fluid retention.[472]

To avoid these far-reaching consequences, testosterone must also be absorbed the skin rather than the stomach. Skin patches and pellet implants have been developed for this purpose. So far, the patches have been manufactured and tested in dosages for men.[473] Studies have not been performed that would establish concentration levels that are suitable for women. Doctors attempting to use them for their female patients can only provide the necessarily lower dosages by trial and error.

As mentioned in previous chapters, implanted pellets were the only route for delivery of estrogen and testosterone I could use successfully. Even though this technology appears to be more commonplace in Europe, in America they are not always covered by some insurance companies because they are still not FDA approved. Since they require approximately 2 to 3 office visits a year, at a cost of between $200 and $300 for each implanting, which may not always be reimbursable, this method could become a personal financial burden.

Finding Hormone Replacement That Works

Women's Normal Hormone Ranges

Artificial hormone replacement runs into additional problems because every women has her own individualized levels.[474] As indicated below, there is a very wide range which is considered normal for each hormone (depending on the day of a woman's monthly cycle).

Table 9	**Normal Hormone Ranges**		
Estrogen:	61	- 437.0	pg/ml[a]
Progesterone:	<1.4	- 23.0	ng/ml[b]
Testosterone:	20	- 120.0	ng%[c]

(a) picograms/milliliter
(b) nanograms/milliliter
(c) nanograms percent

Source: Westcliff Medical Laboratories, Inc.,
Laboratory Test Report Form, Garden Grove, CA.

Since women are not tested before surgery to determine their "normal" levels, they cannot be restored to their unique pre-surgical status. "What was her normal?" It is impossible to know, or to prescribe standard dosages that will work for all women. In attempting to provide women with the same hormonal balance to which their bodies have been accustomed, doctors can only guess and try, and if it doesn't work, guess and try again.

Additionally, tracking the HRT women receive can be difficult. The testing of hormone levels is dependent on the method of detection used, the test equipment, and on the technologist who is performing the test. Send the same blood samples to two different labs, or even the same lab at a later date, and you will get slightly different answers.[475] This lack of consistency, combined with the wide range of normal, makes it difficult to monitor any women on HRT.

Side-effects

Research reveals that side-effects from hormone therapy have caused a number of women to discontinue its use.[476] A major reason for the different side-effects is our incredible individuality. What works for one, may not work for another. However, there are so many types, routes, combinations of delivery throughout the month, and dosages available, women should not give up until they find the combination that suits their own bodies. The benefits to their cardiovascular system and bones will be worth the effort.

Recreating What Surgically Altered Women Have Lost

We need to impress upon pharmaceutical companies the importance of creating safe technologies to deliver hormones in concentrations suitable for all women. Safe routes of delivery must be developed that will not do more harm than good to bodies that have already been compromised.

Today, most of the estrogen patches are manufactured for naturally postmenopausal women and do not meet the additional needs of oophorectomized women. From my own experience, and those of other oophorectomized women, they are not a high enough dosage to eliminate our symptoms. Surgically castrated women need stronger dosages of estrogen, as well as testosterone patches designed for them.

In reality, however, current technology cannot recreate the complexities of the human body. The far-reaching consequences to the liver, alone, demonstrates that no pill can replace what nature so effortlessly produces in our bodies. The few ovarian chemicals that have been identified, and therefore artificially replaced, do not function like those a woman's body manufactures naturally. How can they be regulated to deliver the precise amount of hormones, at the exact appropriate time, with the necessary feedback for the production of more, or less, gradually and precisely every minute of every day, the same as an intact non-surgically altered body? The slow diffusion of the pellets and patches, avoids the sharp spikes and low ebbs of the hormone levels pills create in the blood, making this method of delivery the closest to what nature provides for women. However, nothing artificially manufactured can automatically regulate these hormones according to a woman's own rhythm and balance, like her own body does so beautifully and effortlessly, all by itself. Women's bodies can never be the same as they were before losing their finely tuned, self-regulating organs. It is time to reconsider the practice of all prophylactic oophorectomies, as well as hysterectomies performed for benign reasons.

15

Social, Medical, Political and Economic Institutions: Why Is This Practice so Well Entrenched?

Why is America still performing more hysterectomies than many other countries in the world?

Social

Risk To Life

What is your life worth? A million dollars? What is it worth to live without constant pain, or being dependent on others? Ten million dollars? Only a family who has lost a wife and mother, can answer the first question. Only a woman, bedridden with a broken hip, like Michelle, can answer the second one.

Hysterectomies have been performed in record numbers throughout this entire century. Every year 300 to 1,000 families in America are told their wives or mothers died. For what? These women were not facing any fatal disease. Their condition did not kill them. Surgery did. As many as 40,000 women have died just since 1964 alone. Why have we allowed "standard medical practice" to kill this many women each year? During the Viet Nam War, approximately 55,000 American men were killed. At the time, there were marches and endless debates of public outrage claiming that we were killing off our men needlessly. Where are the outcries about this quiet war that has been legally killing women under the banner of "standard medical practice."

The women in America who have died from the consequences of this surgery represent only a small portion of the total global impact. This number does not include the statistics and rates for the rest of the world, where 70-90% of hysterectomies are also performed for non-life-threatening conditions, nor does it include those who have died from the long-term consequences of surgery. How many have died early in life as a result of coronary disease or osteoporotic breaks, conditions which have not been correlated to their hysterectomies? It is time to look at the true cost this operation has on women's lives.

Risk To Quality Of Life

Doctors do not warn women of the potential problems hysterectomies can create. When problems surface, doctors do not know how to help their patients, so they refer them to psychiatrists. As a result, hysterectomized women's marriages and relationships are torn apart when, neither they, nor the men who love them, understand the changes in mood, emotionality, or sexuality. The world needs to reshape its thinking about childbearing organs before more families are torn apart and jobs are lost, ultimately affecting our whole society.

Alzheimer's Disease

Another critical area needing to be addressed is the research that indicates low estrogen levels may play a role in Alzheimer's disease. Estrogen is being investigated, not only for the fact that women make up the vast majority of those afflicted, but because more and more studies are revealing that several of the critical functions estrogen performs in the brain are also the same areas of deficiencies found in Alzheimer's patients.

Alzheimer's sufferers exhibit two conditions which are associated with low estrogen levels: 1) When Alzheimer's patients are compared to those without disease, they have increased cortisol levels.[477] 2) Additionally, the majority of Alzheimer's patients who demonstrate improved cognitive and emotional functioning in response to estrogen therapy, also have osteoporosis; whereas those patients who do not show an improvement in their testing scores, do not have concomitant osteoporosis.[478] Both of these conditions suggest estrogen deficiency may play a role in the development of Alzheimer's in a subset of patients.

Further verification of this possibility is found in studies on research animals and postmenopausal women. They show estrogen therapy not only increases memory and reasoning ability, but significantly delays the onset or reduces the risk Alzheimer's as well.[479] There are two roles of estrogen that have been identified which could lead to this improved functioning. These functions are increased blood supply to the tissues, and protection of nerve cells.[480]

Women who are expecting a hysterectomy to improve their quality of life should be advised that their ovaries may shut down early, and that the questions surrounding decreased estrogen's possible role in the development and progression of Alzheimer's disease are not resolved. The fact that this is being researched as a possible cause of Alzheimer's makes it even more imperative to stop oophorectomizing women. Until more is known, we should not expose women to more years of estrogen loss.

This has implications, not only for the estimated 4 million Americans who suffer from Alzheimer's, but for our whole nation as well. The average cost per person afflicted with this devastating disease is estimated to be $174,000. The present annual cost of $100 billion, much of it taxpayers, is expected to climb staggeringly as the Baby Boomer generation approaches Medicare age.[481]

Life Style And Diet

One important factor women need to look at is the diet in westernized countries. PMS and menopause symptoms appear to be an accepted fact of life in America and Europe, yet Asian women do not have the same rate of symptoms. Studies show between 60-78% of menopausal age women in westernized countries report hot flushes, as compared to 0-39% in many Asian countries.[482] Even when their ovaries are removed, only 24% of Chinese women in Hong Kong experience hot flushes.[483] This difference extends to other conditions related to menopause, such as osteoporosis, which has a much lower incidence rate in Asia than that found in western countries.

The life style of these countries is considered to be a major contributing factor for these differences. Their rural populations, in particular, experience physical activity and direct exposure to sunlight, and they eat a high proportion of soy products containing phytoestrogens (estrogen-like compounds), green tea, and rice.[484] The combination of diet, weight-bearing exercise, vitamin D manufactured by their bodies from exposure to the sun, along with drinking green tea (which is thought to offer protection from osteoporosis), results in fewer menopausal symptoms and stronger bones.

Articles, citing fear of an alteration in the Asian diet due to increased exposure to westernized countries, urge public health education programs to encourage a retention of their "good life style." This recommendation is being promoted because they know, with their huge population, the financial burden of rampant osteoporosis, alone, could be overwhelming.[485]

Life Style And Cancer

The differences in life styles also reflect drastically different rates in breast cancer. In 1990, statistics show the incidence rate for the development of breast cancer in the United States was 110 per 100,000.[486] This contrasts greatly with the rate in Singapore at the same time, which was 39 per 100,000.[487] Even though this rate was less than half that of the United States, statistics reveal that it doubled in just 20 years, as the rate in 1970 was only 20 per 100,000.[488] Investigations reveal that part of this sharp increase in cancer is strongly associated with their rapid economic progress and urbanization, which has resulted in a diet of higher and excess calorie intake, leading to abdominal obesity for women between 45 to 69 years old.[489]

Other factors appearing to be involved are changes in menstruation and reproduction. These alterations, also resulting from urbanization, include fewer births (each additional delivery results in an 18% decreased of risk of breast cancer), a dropping in age for the start of menstruation, less breast feeding, age at last pregnancy, and age at menopause. Even though all these changes indicate an estrogen involvement, this study also revealed the unexpected finding that women who used, or were using HRT, had a reduced risk of breast cancer, compared with women who had never received HRT.[490] This is yet another study providing conflicting results as to whether estrogen use can lead to breast cancer.

With such a disparity of symptoms and rates of diseases between countries, the critical factor of diet and life style should not be overlooked by America or other countries having high osteoporosis, heart disease, and breast cancer rates, as well as where PMS and menopausal symptoms run rampant.[491]

Medical

Prophylactic Ovarian Removal

Since fear of ovarian cancer is cited as the reason to remove ovaries at the time of a hysterectomy, and there has also been concern that taking estrogens can increase the risk of breast cancer, it behooves women to look at the actual risks of each type of cancer. Breast cancer is so much more common than ovarian cancer, every year 7 times more women are diagnosed, and 3 times more women die from breast cancer than ovarian cancer. Yet, the fear of ovarian cancer has convinced millions of women to give up their ovaries, making them turn to some type of estrogen replacement program to protect their hearts and bones. If the medical community's concern that taking estrogen increases the risk of breast cancer is true, then prophylactic ovarian removal does not make sense. In its attempts to eliminate one cancer, the practice forces women into requiring ongoing estrogen therapy, a therapy which they are also presently theorizing could increase the chance of developing breast cancer, already a seven times greater risk for women. Again, the cure is worse than the disease.

The same prophylactic practice could be advised and promoted for pancreatic cancer. This cancer causes approximately the same number of deaths in women (13,400) as ovarian cancer (13,400).[492] Yet, doctors don't remove everyone's pancreas from fear of cancer, because they know we cannot live without it.

Women's Organs Are Not Expendable

The truth is, women's organs are not expendable either. It just takes longer for the effects of their loss to show up, compared to the pancreas. The changes that occur when women's bodies are deprived of essential chemicals are as silent, and as deadly, as pancreatic or ovarian cancer. The symptoms just take 10, 20, or even 30 years to develop. When the heart attacks, strokes, or osteoporotic hip fractures occur, it is too late to undo the damage created by years of chemical imbalance. The conditions and symptoms resulting from unbalanced hormones are treated individually, without looking into why the body is not working the way it was originally designed, and the connection to a woman's previous hysterectomy is never made. As a result, women do not get the correct medical treatment for the hormone deficiencies which led to these debilitating problems.

Political

Appropriateness Of Hysterectomies

A historic review of this operation provides documented evidence that, as long ago as 1946, hysterectomies were already considered an over-performed operation. When looking at the appropriateness of surgeries at the time, 31% of the patients were found to be free of pathology (no evidence of disease) leading the researcher to state: "But, if what we have observed in this look behind the scenes is confirmed by future studies, then we may be sure that when the curtain rises we shall witness a tragedy, painful and far-reaching in its implications."[493]

Even though the alarms were ringing, it is amazing that the rate of surgeries performed every year was allowed to mushroom to the peak in 1975, when 725,000 women lost these valuable organs.[494] By 1978, hysterectomies were included in a congressional hearing on unnecessary surgeries. The hearing concluded that well over half of the hysterectomies were performed for inappropriate reasons. This shed grave doubts about the validity of the operation, but the call was still not heeded. Today, 20 years later, they are still being performed at a rate of 550,000 annually, with only 10% for life-threatening reasons.

When a quality assurance process was initiated to review a surgeon's indication as to why a hysterectomy was recommended, there was a 24% reduction in the frequency with which the operation was performed.[495] If a hysterectomy had been the only answer, and essential for the well-being of the patient, there would have been no corresponding drop in the numbers when greater scrutiny was placed on the physician's therapeutic recommendation. If second opinions are required, one study showed that in 48% of the cases the consultants did not agree that a hysterectomy was the best therapeutic route.[496]

This evidence of inappropriateness is further confirmed by peer reviews. When doctors evaluated other doctors' decisions as to whether the patient's symptoms and conditions warranted a hysterectomy, 16% of the operations were judged to be an inappropriate route of therapy, with another 25% deemed performed for uncertain reasons.[497]

Economic

Today, economics drives this surgery. It is second only to cesarean section in numbers of operations performed in the United States, generating a revenue of $4 billion for doctors and hospitals every year.

Personal Economic Impact

Hysterectomies create personal economic impact. When

the standard hormone replacement therapies did not work for me, my insurance company would not cover the hormone pellets that did work, because they were not FDA approved. After my auto accident, when my family practitioner ordered routine hormone level checks, the HMO refused to allow them to be performed, stating that they were "not medically indicated." The HMO did not recognize the vital importance of monitoring artificially replaced hormones on a regular basis. As it turned out, this refusal happened to coincide with the beginning of the treatment for my neck injury. If the HMO had approved the hormone level testing at the time, it would have allowed us to detect that I was not absorbing the pellets and saved thousands of dollars spent on therapy my body could not utilize.

Hysterectomized women become high maintenance patients, yet many insurance companies do not recognize their increased needs and problems. In most cases, they will only reimburse what is usual and customary for normal functioning bodies. In attempting to bring my body back to its pre-surgical functioning, extraordinary measures have had to be taken, with the vast majority at my expense. The real cost of my $5,000 one hour operation has exceeded $60,000 in doctors' office visits, hospital stays, extensive therapeutic treatments, prescriptions, food supplement purchases, and gym fees. This does not include time lost from work, or from life itself, as it is impossible to put a price on the years I lost while in the black hole of depression.

Debates Over Which Procedures To Use

Even when faced with the astounding number of complications and deaths originating directly from hysterectomies, the attention has been focused on women's immediate symptoms rather than looking at the best long-term prevention or solutions.

The biggest debates found in the literature have not been whether a hysterectomy is the most beneficial route of therapy for women over their life-time. Instead, more focus has been placed on which method to use in performing the operation. Many studies have been conducted covering the operating room time required, the costs, and the percentage of complications women acquire with each type of surgical procedure.[498]

There are major areas of disagreement over whether the organs should be removed through the vagina or through the abdomen. The current studies show vaginal hysterectomies average $5,200, as compared to the more major abdominal surgery averaging $6,400.[499] The choice of the vaginal route fuels the debate over whether to use a laparoscope (instrument allowing physician to see inside abdominal cavity) to provide a better view for this route of surgery. Utilizing a laparoscope doubles the cost, increasing it to approximately $12,000 per operation (1988 - 1994 estimates).[500]

Insurance companies support these types of studies because their major concern is, "What does it cost today?" Yet, the studies which need to be initiated are the ones that look at the full impact of hysterectomies on a woman's body, her life, and the resultant quality of that life, not on how quickly or cost-effectively her organs can be removed from her body.

With the economic crisis occurring in medicine today, decisions about which types of procedures can, or cannot, be performed may no longer be in the hands of the doctor, or even the patient. Indeed, one researcher stated: "Considering the present attention given to health care costs, it is unknown how much longer physicians will have the luxury of selecting procedures independent of economic influences."[501]

Hospitals and insurance companies look at a hysterectomy as a cost-effective procedure. Since a hysterectomy takes only about an hour, the operating room becomes available for other operations to be performed. Myomectomies (a surgical procedure which saves the uterus by removing just the fibroid tumor) can take 2 to 3 hours, or longer, because of the process of preserving the blood vessels and nerves that supply the uterus. Hospitals may turn down doctors requests for the extra hours of operating room time it may take to save the uterus. As a result, women may no longer have the choice of whether, or not, their organs will be saved.

Health Maintenance Organizations (HMOs) came into being with the concept of providing the physicals and tests needed to maintain one's long-term health. The concept was to save total dollars spent over the life-time of the individual. Yet now, they have established an assembly line procedure that leads women with gynecological problems right into operating rooms for hysterectomies. The medical community and insurance companies do not see that the true long-term cost of removing these organs is far greater than the additional time it takes to save them.

Hysterectomies' True Impact

When hysterectomies became an answer to female problems, doctors believed that the only functions of the uterus and ovaries were childbearing. Medical science had not yet identified the multitude of chemicals produced by these organs, nor the vital, beautifully choreographed, interrelated functions they perform. No studies had been performed to look at the overall, long-term effect hysterectomies have on the body, so the critical roles of the reproductive organs were not known.

Since hysterectomies can impact every bodily system, even though some seem very remote, all future research studies on women, for any condition, should include the information about whether, or not, they have had a hysterectomy. Even then, it will be hard to get clear-cut, unbiased results, because of variations between women, whether their ovaries were removed or not, or if they were damaged by the surgery. However, only these types of studies will bring awareness to hysterectomies' true impact, and help show that women cannot live long, healthy, independent lives without their reproductive organs intact.

National Economic Impact

The $4,000 to $12,000 for the initial surgery is only the beginning of the cost. In reality, the lifetime after-care cost is in the 10s of billions of dollars. Just osteoporosis alone, one of the major outcomes of the surgery, costs Americans between $10 and $18 billion a year.

The tremendous numbers of surgeries performed has resulted in 25% of American women undergoing a hysterectomy by the age of 60. Since the long-term consequences do not show up until years later, by the time the medical conditions do appear, these women are of Medicare age. The national health care system inherits these problems, with tax payers ultimately paying the bill. With the Social Security system (Medicare) projecting bankruptcy, America cannot afford to keep stripping over 1/2 million women a year of these health maintaining organs.

The new Medicare appropriation legislation is including mandatory funding for bone-density scans for all women without ovaries, due to their high risk for osteoporosis. This is the beginning, not only of acknowledging the true consequences of ovarian removal, but also to the awareness of what the resultant osteoporosis truly costs the American public.

In our age, every dollar is important to the already overburdened government, medical system, insurance companies, HMO's, and health care plans. So, why are we blindly willing to add the needless cost of hysterectomizing and prophylactically ovariectomizing millions of women to our society? It is time to acknowledge that some of the nation's burgeoning medical crisis is due in part to the epidemic of hysterectomy and oophorectomy surgeries performed over the last 50 years. Billions of dollars are being spent trying to fix what has been destroyed. We can no longer afford to ignore the long-term effects that result from depletion of the body's essential hormones and chemicals produced by women's childbearing organs.

16

Whole Body = Whole Functioning

America became rich and famous by developing the assembly line. The process made it cost-effective to reproduce the same results, consistently. This same thinking has left us with the concept that everybody is the same and can be treated like an assembly line. Women are not identical and they cannot all be treated alike. Their individual uniqueness is what causes the varied reactions to hysterectomies which have constantly perplexed doctors. First, some women feel fine, while others are sent into the depths of hell. Second, not all women experience relief from the symptoms that led them to a hysterectomy in the first place. Third, they may trade their non-life-threatening conditions for potential death, both immediately (there is no surgery which does not have the risk of death connected to it), or later, due to the silent diseases created by the disruption of their finely tuned hormone and chemical balance.

Hormones are not only essential in controlling and integrating reproduction, they also maintain the body's entire metabolism and balance. One physiology textbook states that we could function without our hormones, but: ". . . life would be extremely precarious and abnormal; individuals would be unable to adapt to environmental alteration or stress, and their physical and mental abilities would be drastically impaired. They would require the constant attention bestowed upon a hothouse plant."[502]

The human body is very complex. There are so many intricately interrelated hormones, it is almost impossible to determine the total effect the loss of ovarian or uterine chemicals may have throughout the body. Researchers have a difficult time isolating how the altering of even one chemical affects the whole system. To understand this complexity, picture the researchers in the center of a circle of 100 television sets all tuned to different channels. When one channel changes, all 100 pictures change simultaneously. Since it is impossible to see all the sets at the same time, there is no way to determine the domino effect that one change created.

It is just as impossible to see all the changes hysterectomies create in the body, nor do we have the technology to measure them all. This is one reason why studies, in every area of investigation on the effect of hysterectomies, give conflicting and sometimes completely opposite results.

However, what IS clear: the delicate, extremely complex hormonal balance of the body is disrupted by the removal of the reproductive organs, and the medical community really does not know the full extent of the changes hysterectomies and oophorectomies inflict on women's bodies. What is disrupted, the full extent of that disruption to the rest of the body, and how to recreate the body's precisely choreographed rhythm remains mostly unknown. Many research studies end by stating that they do not know how it all works. Until studies all give the same definitive answers, it is imperative to stop the mass removal of organs that are so important and life-preserving for women.

Everyone needs to recognize that the loss of a woman's uterus and ovaries can be lethal. It is so much more complex than just replacing estrogen, progesterone, and testosterone.

Removal of these organs creates holes in the body's interrelated, synergistic, complex chemical systems. Artificial replacement of only a few of the many expertly tuned hormones and chemicals that women lose, when their God-given organs are cut out, can never equal how eloquently nature designed their bodies to function.

Hysterectomized And Oophorectomized Women

All women who have had a hysterectomy and/or oophorectomy, even though they may not show symptoms today, need to start taking care of their bodies to counteract the silent conditions presented in this book. Compared to naturally menopausal women, it is even more critical for them to maintain a diet and an exercise program that preserves their bones, as well as protects their cardiovascular system. In addition, routine physical exams monitoring cholesterol and LDL/HDL ratios, blood pressure, and bone densities will help reveal changes early enough to start taking more aggressive steps to counteract them.

Women Facing The Hysterectomy Decision

Women, who are facing the decision of having a hysterectomy, need to understand that the human body was not designed to function with critical pieces missing. Removal of organs can create more problems for them in the future than the ones they are currently experiencing, affecting their bodies' biochemistry, and ultimately their quality of life, forever.

All the potential consequences discussed in this book are real. These long-term effects may seem so remote, or so far in the future they can make women feel, "Who, me?" . . . "It won't happen to me." It **HAS** happened to millions of women who are left having to take time-consuming and exorbitantly costly care of themselves for the rest of their lives.

I have written this book wanting every woman to realize the serious consequences which can occur when their reproductive organs are removed, and understand the futility of our medical community in attempting to recreate the many functions the uterus and ovaries automatically perform in their bodies. The documentation clearly proves that it is not a question of whether, or not, a woman's body will be irreparably damaged, but rather: <u>WHEN will the symptoms start to show</u>? These are the realities. Why trade today's symptoms for a greater chance of heart disease, death, paralysis from stroke, depression, Alzheimer's disease, or possible loss of sexual enjoyment for the rest of your life? Why trade treatable symptoms for trial and error artificial hormone replacement, necessitating being under a doctor's care for continual monitoring and laboratory testing. Why be subjected to the side-effects from medications? Why risk winding up in a nursing home with an unmendable broken hip due to osteoporosis?

Alternatives

All women, when faced with the decision of "electing" to have their vital organs removed, deserve to be empowered to make a truly informed, educated choice. Are these risks worth it? In my case, absolutely not. If, prior to my surgery, someone had relayed to me the information embodied in this book, I know I would not have submitted my body to the loss of these vital organs. Most of the women now considering elective hysterectomies can be helped in other ways. Today, there are alternatives for every condition, even some cancers, for which hysterectomies have been recommended as the best answer in the past. New techniques have come to the forefront that resolve many troublesome female problems; solutions which do not set up a potential for a lifetime of the difficult consequences that can result from removing women's valuable childbearing organs.

Books are listed in the appendix that cover alternatives for heavy bleeding, fibroids, ovarian cysts, and endometriosis. These alternatives do not sentence women to the slow, inevitable fat build-up in their arteries, and the daily loss of bone that results from removing their natural estrogen protection and other vital chemicals 10 to 30 years earlier than normal.

Please educate yourselves about all these alternatives. Find a doctor who is willing to use alternative therapies so that, together, you can decide which is the best course of action. For myself, I wish I had had the opportunity to read the following conclusion before I made my decision: "Very, very few patients should ever have a hysterectomy just because of bleeding. That is an endocrine (hormone) disease largely, and in most instances it can be treated medically and not surgically."[503] Today's therapies can alleviate your current problem, while saving your organs, allowing you to stay the whole functioning human being God intended everyone to be.

We and our medical providers, together, need to switch our focus from one of fear, to one of love. The practice of hysterectomies has been allowed to escalate to epidemic proportions out of fear of cancer and out of ignorance about how our body is an integrated whole; one which is not nearly as functional with pieces missing. Operating out of fear has permitted valuable pieces of a wondrously intricate puzzle to be cut away, sentencing women's bodies to never work the same way again. It is time to honor our bodies and the beautiful way they were created to work in such incredibly complex harmony. The body is awesomely designed to heal itself, and we should work with techniques that allow the <u>whole</u> body to heal back to wellness.

In 1976 two researchers wrote: "An operation that results in complications for 30 to 45 of every 100 women receiving it, and is followed by death in one woman in 500 to 1,000, can be considered to have considerable somatic (bodily) impact that can have major psychological reactions. Yet on the level of pure cultural patterning, hysterectomy has become so common it is seen as almost 'normal.' Such widespread acceptance may tend to mute the recognition of not only the physical but also the psychosomatic and social sequelae (complications that follow)."[504] It is time to recognize that this practice is not "normal" for the human body.

Now, with this much biochemical proof, it behooves all of us, women and doctors alike, to change our beliefs about elective organ removal. Medical dictates have been wrong in the past. Blood letting, a "standard medical practice" for over two hundred years, sped many people, including George Washington, to their deaths. Today, we wonder how anyone could possibly think patients were being helped with such erroneous reasoning. As the information provided in this book becomes accepted common knowledge, future generations will be just as incredulous about our current "standard medical practice" of hysterectomizing over 1/2 million women every year.[505]

If I save one woman's life, my experience and the writing of this book will have been worth it. My goal, though, is to enlighten millions of women as to the potential devastation their bodies can undergo.

Don't play Russian Roulette with your life, or the quality of that life.

"Elizabeth, . . . Elizabeth, . . .

you have to wake up women,

everywhere."

Epilogue

At publication time, I am still struggling with finding a satisfactory route of HRT. The pellets, which worked the best for me, are difficult to obtain here in America.

My research revealed that doctors do have to perform the prophylactic resewing of the vagina (medically termed a colporrhaphy) at the time of surgery. This is done to prevent the vaginal prolapse that hysterectomies would otherwise cause a large percentage of the time. The numbness and my inability to control my vagina muscles did go away, although it took years for the nerves to regrow.

Fibromyalgia symptoms, as well as hot flushes, appear very quickly when my estrogen replacement drops in any way. Acupuncture provided the best sleep I had experienced in years, and Chinese herbs have helped me feel more comfortable.

Presently, I am not on blood pressure medication. The Chinese acupressure technique of Jin Shin Do worked the best in bringing it under control on a day to day basis. Under stress, however, without the uterine and ovarian chemicals which work to maintain balance, it still skyrockets immediately. My cholesterol has remained steady at 230, so I have no answers as yet on how to lower it.

My abdominal pain finally did disappear, but not for several years after the surgery.

Not every therapy works for all, ultimately every woman has to experiment to determine which therapeutic techniques work best for her.

Sadly, I wish I didn't have to struggle with any of these conditions. Women, please honor your bodies; don't subject yourselves to having to live with any of these known, or unknown possibilities.

To the Reader

Elizabeth is interested in hearing your personal experiences regarding these subjects. Please contact her via the Internet, e-mail, or write to her in care of New Voice Publications.

World wide web:	www.newvoice.**net**
e-mail:	elizabeth@newvoice.**net**
Mailing address:	New Voice Publications P. O. Box 14133 Irvine, CA 92623-4133
To order the book:	800 Booklog (800 266-5564) or at www.newvoice.**net**

Reading List

Anatomy of the Spirit, by Caroline Myss, Ph.D., Random House, 1996.

Estrogen, by Lila E. Nachtigall, M.D. and Joan Rattner Heilman, HarperPerennial, 1991.

Health, Happiness & Hormones: One Woman's Journey Toward Health After A Hysterectomy, by Arlene Swaney, Starburst, 1996.

The Hysterectomy Hoax, by Stanley West, M.D., Doubleday, 1994.

I'm Too Young To Get Old, by Judith Reichman, M.D., Random House, 1996.

The No-Hysterectomy Option: Your Body-Your Choice, by Herbert A. Goldfarb, M.D., John Wiley & Sons, 1990.

No More Hysterectomies, by Vickie Hufnagel, M.D., NAL Penguin, 1988.

Quantum Healing, by Deepak Chopra, M.D., Bantam Book, 1989..

Women's Bodies, Women's Wisdom, by Christiane Northrup, M.D., Bantam Books, 1994.

You Don't Need A Hysterectomy: New and Effective Ways of Avoiding Major Surgery, by Ivan Strausz, M.D., Addison-Wesley Publishing Group, 1993.

List of Abbreviations

5-HT: serotonin

5-HT$_{2A}$: area of the brain known as 5-HT$_{2A}$

ACTH: adrenocorticotropic hormone

CAD: coronary artery disease

CDC: Centers for Disease Control (U.S.)

CHD: coronary heart disease

FSH: follicle stimulating hormone

GH: growth hormone

GTT: glucose tolerance tests

HDL: high-density-lipoproteins

HMO: Health Management Organization

HPA or HPA axis: hypothalamus-pituitary-adrenal glands

HRT: hormone replacement therapy

IC: interstitial cystitis

ICU: Intensive Care Unit

IR: insulin resistance

LDL: low-density-lipoproteins

M.A. : Master of Arts Degree

MAO: monamine oxidase

M.T. : Licensed Medical Technologist

NIDDM: non-insulin-dependent diabetes mellitus

PDR: *Physician's Desk Reference*

PG's: prostaglandins

REM: sleep characterized by rapid eye movement

SHBG: sex hormone binding globulin

TSH: thyroid stimulating hormone

USO: unilateral-salpingo-oophorectomy

VLDL: very-low-density-lipoproteins

Glossary

5-HT: see serotonin.

5-HT$_{2A}$: an area of the brain which controls mood, mental state, cognition, emotion, and behavior.

17β-estradiol: (also known as **17beta-estradiol**) one of the group of estrogens manufactured in body. It is the predominant form found in the body before menopause, manufactured primarily in the ovaries.

Abdominal hysterectomy: removal of the uterus through a cut in the abdominal wall.

ACTH: see adrenocorticotropic hormone.

Adrenocorticotropic hormone (ACTH): a hormone secreted by the pituitary gland which stimulates the adrenal cortex to secret its entire spectrum of hormones.

Alzheimer's disease: a form of brain disease. It can lead to confusion, memory loss, restlessness, problems with perception, speech trouble, trouble moving, and fearing things that are not there. Breakdown of the cells of the brain does occur.

Androgens: any steroid hormone that promotes the development and maintenance of male or masculine characteristics, present in both men and women.

Angiotensin: see renin-angiotensin.

Antidepressant: any drug used to alleviate depression by altering chemicals in the brain.

Arteriosclerosis: degenerative changes in arteries which result in thickening of the walls, and loss of elasticity, and sometimes calcium deposits.

Atherosclerosis: changes to the inside lining of arteries by the accumulation of lipids (fats), complex carbohydrates, blood and blood products, fibrous tissue, and calcium deposits. These plaque formations are major causes of heart disease, chest pain (angina), heart attacks, and other disorders of the circulation.

Beta-endorphins: a form of endorphin, see endorphins.

Bilateral oophorectomy (BSO): removal of both ovaries.

Bile: a fluid secreted by the liver, sorted in the gallbladder and released for the digestion of fat.

Blood platelets: see platelets.

CAD: see coronary artery disease.

Calcitonin: a thyroid hormone which plays an essential role in bone metabolism, by inhibiting bone resorption (breakdown). Its secretion is influenced by the amount of calcium in the blood.

Carcinoma: cancer.

Castration: the removal of one or both ovaries or testicles.

Cervix: the lower portion, or neck of the uterus.

Cholesterol: an essential component in the formation of the cell membrane, and in several hormones, such as testosterone and estrogen. Cholesterol is manufactured by the body and is also found in the animal foods we eat. A large part of most gallstones, it occurs in plaques in the arteries, in various cysts, and in cancerous tissue.

Clitoris: the erogenous small cylindrical erectile structure in the female, which corresponds to the male penis.

Colorectal functioning: of, or pertaining to the actions of the colon and rectum.

Connective tissue: tissue that support and joins other body tissue and parts. It also carries materials for processing, nutrition, and waste release. Examples are bone, cartilage, and fibrous connective tissue.

Constrict: tightening, or contracting, or narrowing.

Coronary artery disease (CAD): any abnormal condition that may affect the arteries of the heart. The most common kind is atherosclerosis.

Corticoid-steroids: any of the steroids made in the adrenal cortex which are chiefly involved in carbohydrate, fat, and protein metabolism, or in the regulation of electrolyte and water balance. They are used clinically for hormone replacement therapy, as anti-inflammatory agents, and to suppress the immune response.

Cortisol: made by the adrenal cortex, it is the major natural hormone which affects the metabolism of glucose, protein, and fats. It also regulates the immune system. Hydrocortisone is the form used in treatment.

Diabetes: a disease affecting sugar use by the body.

Diastolic blood pressure: the lowest blood pressure reading, which occurs between the heart's contractions.

Dilate: see dilation.

Dilation: to undergo physiological or artificial enlargement of a hollow structure or opening. The act of stretching or enlarging. To enlarge, expand, relax, or open.

Dysfunction: disturbance, impairment, or abnormality of the functioning of a body organ or system.

Eclampsia: convulsions or seizures associated with pregnancy. Associated with high blood pressure, it is the gravest form of poisoning of pregnancy.

Endocrine (organ) gland: a ductless gland that releases hormones directly into the blood. They affect the function of specific target organs and exert powerful influences on growth, sexual development, and metabolism.

Endometrial cancer: cancer of the lining of the uterus.

Endometriosis: the abnormal occurrence of tissue which resembles the endometrium (lining of the uterus) in various locations in the pelvic cavity, including the uterine wall, ovaries, or extragenital sites.

Endorphins: substances that bind to opiate receptors in various areas of the brain, one function appears to be to raise the pain threshold.

Enzyme: a protein that speeds up, or causes chemical reactions in living matter.

Estrogen receptor: see receptor.

Estrogen (oestrogen): female hormone produced by the ovaries, responsible for female sexual characteristics.

Estrone: one of the group of estrogens manufactured in body. It is the predominant form found in the body after menopause, manufactured primarily in the fat tissue.

Fasting: to abstain from eating for 8 hours or more before the drawing of blood for specific laboratory tests.

Fecal incontinence: see incontinence.

Fibrinogen: one of the primary proteins necessary for the formation of blood clots in the body.

Fibroid tumors: see fibroids.

Fibroids: (fibroid tumors/leiomyomata/myomata) benign tumors which stem from the smooth muscle of the uterus. A common cause for heavy bleeding in women.

Fibromyalgia: a syndrome whose symptoms include widespread muscle pain, persistent fatigue, generalized morning stiffness, multiple tender points, and non-refreshing sleep.

Flushes: see hot flushes

Frankenhauser's plexus: the lower portion of a large nerve complex that connects to the ureters, bladder, rectum, uterus, and vagina, which can be damaged during pelvic surgery.

GH: see growth hormone.

Glucose tolerance test (GTT): a test of the body's ability to process carbohydrates as well as its insulin response. Utilized in the diagnosis of diabetes, it is performed by giving a dose of glucose (sugar) and then measuring the blood and urine for glucose.

Gonadal (sex) hormones: chemicals secreted by the female or male sex glands; ovaries or testicles.

Growth hormone (GH): a substance released by the pituitary gland which promotes protein (muscle) building, utilization of fat for energy, and reduces use of carbohydrates.

Gynecologist: physician specializing in the care and treatment of women and their diseases, especially those affecting the sexual organs.

HDL: see high density lipoprotein.

High density lipoprotein (HDL): the smallest, most dense lipoprotein (fat) in the blood. It beneficially performs the role of pulling cholesterol out of the body by transporting it to the liver for removal.

HMO: Health Management Organization; these provide managed health care for groups.

Hormone: a chemical messenger substance produced in organs of the body, transported by the blood, and having a specific regulatory effect on the activity of certain cells or organs remote from its origin.

Hot flashes: see hot flushes.

Hot flushes: also called hot flashes, temporary rises in body temperature associated with menopause.

HPA axis: see hypothalamus-pituitary-adrenal glands.

HRT: see hormone replacement therapy.

Hypertension: the medical term for high blood pressure.

Hypothalamus-pituitary-adrenal axis (HPA axis): many integrated functions of the body are regulated by the complex interactions performed by the secretion of hormones from the hypothalamus, pituitary gland, and adrenal glands. They play key roles in: the body's reaction to stress, immune and anti-inflammatory responses, regulation of carbohydrate metabolism, cardiovascular system, electrolyte balance; and the central nervous system, influencing behavior, mood, excitability, and electrical activity of neurons.

Hypothalamus: region of the brain below the thalamus, which, with the pituitary, regulates internal organs.

Hysterectomy: surgical removal of the uterus.

IC: see interstitial cystitis.

Impaired Glucose Tolerance: when GTT values fall in between a normal response and a full diabetic condition. It indicates that the individual is developing insulin resistance. Investigators have identified that a subgroup of genetically predisposed individuals, who evolve into the non-insulin-dependent type of diabetes (known as NIDDM), begin with insulin resistance.

Incontinence: the inability or failure to hold or control one's urine or feces.

Insulin resistance (IR): a subnormal response to insulin, identified by GTT values which fall in between a normal response and a full diabetic condition.

Insulin: protein hormone made by the islets of Langerhans in the pancreas. It participates, together with other chemicals, in regulating carbohydrate and fat metabolism. It checks the accumulation of glucose in the blood and promotes the utilization of sugar in the treatment of diabetes.

Interstitial cystitis (IC): a bladder inflammation, characterized by inflamed, ulcerated, and scarred bladder wall, which occurs almost exclusively in women; producing symptoms similar to urinary infection, including urinary urgency, day and night frequency, and pain.

IR: see insulin resistance.

Irritable bowel syndrome (IBS): abnormally increased motility of small and large intestines, accompanied by pain and diarrhea.

Laparoscope: a long slender instrument used for the visual examination of the interior of a body cavity.

Laparoscopic hysterectomy: a procedure for removing the uterus with the aid of a laparoscope.

LDL/HDL ratio: ratio of unhealthy to healthy fats in the blood, monitored to reduce the risk of cardiovascular disease.

LDL: see low-density-lipoprotein.

Leiomyoma/leiomyomas/leiomyomata: see fibroids.

Lipids: any one of a group of fats or fat-like substances. Technically, it is a general term for a number of different water-insoluble compounds found in the body.

Lipoproteins: molecules that contain varying proportions of protein and fats, which are the primary transporters of fats and cholesterol within the bloodstream.

Low-density-lipoprotein: intermediate in size and density between high density lipoproteins (HDL) and very low density lipoproteins (VLDL). It transports cholesterol to body tissues.

MAO (monamine oxidase): an enzyme, found within cells of most tissues, that breaks down many nervous system chemicals, such as serotonin.

MAO inhibition/inhibitors: any drug that stops the action of monamine oxidase (MAO) from breaking down chemicals, particularly serotonin. The drugs are used mainly in the treatment of depression, due to their ability to preserve higher levels of serotonin in the bloodstream.

Menopause: physical loss of menstruation (periods), either as a normal part of aging around the average age of 51, or as a result of surgery.

Menstrual cycle: a woman's monthly reproductive cycle.

Menstruation: that part of a woman's menstrual cycle when the superficial two-thirds of the endometrium is almost all shed as part of the menstrual flow.

Metabolism: the sum of all the chemical processes that take place in the body involving the movement of nutrients in the blood after digestion, resulting in growth, energy, release of waste, and other body functions.

Morbidity: the frequency of the occurrence of complications following a surgical procedure or treatment. An abnormal diseased state or condition.

Mortality: a fatal outcome, or death.

Myoma/myomas/myomata: a benign tumor made of muscular fiber in the uterus, also see fibroids.

Myomata: plural form of myoma.

Myomectomy: surgical removal of a myoma or myomata, or uterine fibroids, while preserving the uterus.

Nardil®: a monoamine oxidase inhibitor, used as an antidepressant.

Nerve growth factor (NGF): a protein produced by the body with hormone-like action that affects the growth and care of nerve cells.

Neurotransmitter: any chemical that changes or results in the sending of nerve signals across spaces separating nerve fibers. They are the essential substances nerves use to convey their messages to cells, enabling the body to respond accordingly.

NGF: see nerve growth factor.

NIDDM: see non-insulin-dependent diabetes mellitus.

Non-insulin-dependent diabetes mellitus (NIDDM): type II diabetes mellitus. An often mild form of diabetes of gradual onset with minimal and no symptoms of metabolic disturbance, with no requirement for insulin. Peak age of onset is 50 to 60 years. Obesity and possibly a genetic factor are usually present.

Oestrogen: see estrogen.

Oophorectomy: surgery to remove one or both of the ovaries. Also known as ovariectomy or castration.

Oophorohysterectomy: the surgical removal of the ovaries and uterus.

Osteoblasts: cells that bring together the substances that form new bone.

Osteoporosis: a decrease in bone tissue with a reduction in bone mass along with increased interior space (small holes), resulting in thinning, demineralization, and weakening of the bones, making them more vulnerable to breakage from minimal trauma; sometimes accompanied by pain or body deformity.

Ovarian cyst: a small sack filled with fluid or semisolid material that grows in or on the ovary.

Ovariectomy: see oophorectomy.

Ovaries: the female gonads or reproductive glands, that correspond to the male testicles. Their function is to store and release eggs and to manufacture hormones.

Pancreas: a gland that produces insulin and chemicals that are involved in the metabolism of glucose (sugar).

Pap smear: test used as a screening for cervical cancer and can also detect vaginal cancer.

Parathyroid gland: a gland next to the thyroid that secretes the parathyroid hormone. Also see parathyroid hormone.

Parathyroid hormone: a hormone secreted by the parathyroid gland, which helps maintain normal calcium levels in the bloodstream. This action in turn keeps the muscle tone, blood clotting, and cell membranes normal.

Parnate®: monoamine oxidase inhibitor, used as an antidepressant.

Partial hysterectomy: see subtotal hysterectomy.

Phospholipids: any fat that contains phosphorous. The major form of lipid (fat) in all cell membranes.

Pituitary gland: small endocrine gland situated at the base of the brain, which secretes many hormones that regulate growth and metabolism.

Placebo: an inactive substance give as if it were a real dose of a needed drug. They are used in drug studies to compare the effects of the inactive substance with those of an experimental drug.

Plaque: a patch of fatty buildup on the lining of a blood vessel. Atherosclerosis of the arteries.

Plasma: the liquid part of the blood.

Platelets: small disc shaped structures in the bloodstream which play a critical role in clotting of the blood.

PMS: see premenstrual syndrome.

Postmenopausal: occurring after the menopause.

Premarin®: a brand name for conjugated equine estrogens collected from pregnant mares' urine, chiefly in the form of estrone sulfate.

Premenopausal: occurring before the menopause.

Premenstrual syndrome (PMS): the diagnostic term used to describe a variety of physical, psychological, and emotional symptoms occurring just prior to menstrual flow (periods).

Progesterone receptor: see receptor.

Progesterone: a steroid hormone produced by the ovary after ovulation takes place which prepares the uterus for implantation of a fertilized ovum (egg). It is essential for pregnancy, during which time it reaches levels 300 times normal. It is utilized in HRT and in the management of various ovarian disorders; excessive bleeding, amenorrhea (lack of periods), etc.

Progestin: synthetic or naturally occurring hormone with progesterone-like effects, which produces changes in the uteral endometrium (lining of uterus). Synthetic forms produce biological responses which are different than natural progesterone. One primary utilization is in birth control pills.

Progestogen: a term applied to any substance possessing progesterone-like activity: either natural progesterone, or a modified form having similar actions (synthetic progesterone).

Prolapsed uterus: see uterine prolapse.

Prophylactic ovarian removal: the surgical removal of the ovaries utilized as a preventive measure against possible cancer.

Prophylactic: a procedure that prevents or helps to prevent the development of disease.

Prorenin: the inactive precursor of renin, see renin-angiotensin.

Prostacyclin: prostaglandin I_2; a powerful vasodilator and potent natural inhibitor of platelet aggregation.

Prostaglandins: any of a group of naturally-occurring hydroxy fatty acids that stimulate contractility of the uterus and other smooth muscles. They have the ability to lower blood pressure, regulate acid secretion of the stomach, regulate temperature and platelet aggregation, and control inflammation. They also affect the action of certain hormones.

Prozac®: the brand name of fluoxetine, an antidepressant which works by increasing available serotonin levels.

Receptor: a structure within a cell or on the surface which selectively binds a specific substance (e.g., estrogen, progesterone, testosterone, etc.), the binding of which creates a specific physiologic effect.

REM: that sleep phase of which is characterized by rapid eye movement.

Renin-angiotensin: renin and angiotensin are part of a complex hormone system that plays a primary role in maintaining normal blood pressure throughout the body. These hormones exert profound effects on blood pressure by affecting how much blood vessels constrict. Originally, physiologists thought the hormones and chemicals involved with this system were produced only in the liver and kidneys, but it is now well established that they are also found in the uterus, as well as the ovaries and testicles.

Renin: see renin-angiotensin.

Reproductive organs: the male and female sex glands. In women these include the ovaries, fallopian tubes and uterus.

Resorption: the loss of tissue, such as bone by the breakdown of the tissue, which is soaked up by the blood. The loss of bone by demineralization, or disintegration.

Serotonin (5-HT): a brain neurotransmitter produced from tryptophan with multiple biologic effects in the body, including regulation of sleep, body temperature, blood pressure, learning, appetite, intestinal motility, pain perception, and sexual behavior, as well as reduces the breakdown of collagen. Increasing its level is the basis of antidepressant therapy. Also called 5-HT, or 5-hydroxytryptamine.

Sex hormone binding globulin (SHBG): also known as testosterone-estrogen-binding globulin; a protein that is capable of binding estradiol and testosterone to carry these sex hormones through the bloodstream.

SHBG: see sex hormone binding globulin.

Slow gut transit constipation (STC): persistently reduced bowel frequency.

STC: see slow gut transit constipation.

Substance P: one of most potent vasodilators known. Present in nerve cells throughout the body, it increases contractions of the GI tract, and plays a role in mediating pain, touch, and temperature.

Subtotal hysterectomy: the surgical removal of the body of the uterus, leaving the cervix in place.

Supracervical hysterectomy: see subtotal hysterectomy.

Supravaginal hysterectomy: see subtotal hysterectomy.

Surgical menopause: technically, the removal of the ovaries (oophorectomy or castration); but also sometimes used to refer to the removal of the uterus.

Systolic blood pressure: a measurement which reflects the heart's force at its maximum contraction. In blood pressure readings, the higher of the two measurements.

Testosterone receptor: see receptor.

Testosterone: the major androgenic hormone associated with male secondary sexual characteristics; produced by the testicles and ovaries, as well as the adrenal glands.

Thyroid hormone: hormones produced and released by the thyroid gland, see thyroid.

Thyroid stimulating hormone (TSH): thyroid stimulating hormone (TSH) is a hormone produced and released by the pituitary gland. It travels to the thyroid gland and stimulates the production of the thyroid hormones. It is one the hormones monitored to assess how the thyroid gland is functioning. Estrogen is known to enhance the response of this hormone.

Thyroid: endocrine gland located at the neck just below the larynx, extending around the front and to either side of the trachea (windpipe) and secreting the hormones thyroxine (T4), and triiodothyronine (T3), both vital to growth and metabolism.

Total hysterectomy: the surgical removal of both the cervix and the body of the uterus at the same time.

Tryptophan: an essential dietary amino acid, which is converted in the brain into serotonin.

TSH: see thyroid stimulating hormone.

Tubal ligation: also called tubal sterilization. Involves the blocking of the fallopian tubes as a means of birth-control. There are different methods. Early methods involved cutting, tying, and burning of the tubes; more recent methods include microsurgery and clipping the tubes.

Unilateral-salpingo-oophorectomy (USO): one ovary removed.

USO: see unilateral-salpingo-oophorectomy.

Ureter: one of a pair of tubes that carry urine from the kidneys into the bladder.

Ureteral: of, or pertaining to the ureter.

Urethra: small tubular structure that drains urine from the bladder.

Urethral: of, or pertaining to the urethra.

Urinary incontinence: difficulty in retaining urine, see incontinence.

Uterine prolapse: the falling down of the uterus in varying degrees; from the cervix being within the vaginal cavity, to the entire uterus outside the vagina.

Uterus: the womb of a woman. A pear-shaped hollow, thick-walled muscular organ that houses the developing fetus. It is becoming recognized as an endocrine (hormone) producing organ.

Vagina: a muscular tube about three inches long connecting the uterine cervix with the external female genitals.

Vaginal hysterectomy: removal of the uterus through the vagina without cutting the wall of the abdomen.

Vaginal prolapse: the falling of the vagina, which can lead to its outward protrusion.

Vaginal: of, or pertaining to the vagina.

Vasoconstrictor: any substance that narrows the interior diameter of the blood vessels.

Vasodilation: enlargement of the interior opening of the blood vessels.

Vasodilator: any substance that expands the interior diameter of the blood vessels, see also dilation.

Very-low-density-lipoprotein (VLDL): the largest and least dense lipoprotein. Manufactured in the liver, it transports triglycerides in the bloodstream. See also lipoprotein.

VLDL+LDL/HDL ratio: see LDL/HDL ratio.

VLDL: see very-low-density-lipoprotein.

Notes

Introduction

1   **National Center for Health Statistics: Utilization of short-stay hospitals:**
    Annual summary for the United States.
    In: *Vital & Health Statistics*. Washington, DC. Multiple years 1973-94. Series
    13, numbers 24,26,31,37,41,60,61,64,72,78,
    83,84,91,96,99,106,109,112,119,121,&128.
    Savage W.
    Hysterectomy and sterilisaton rates: regional variations.
    Practitioner. 1983 May. 227:839-845.
    Opit LJ, Hobbs MST.
    Epidemics of procedures: growth in admissions to hospital in western
    Australia, 1972 to 1977.
    Med Jour Aust. 1979 Oct 6. 2:378-380.

2   Lepine LA, Hillis SD, Marchbanks PA, et al.
    Hysterectomy surveillance—United States, 1980 -1993.
    MMWR, Center For Disease Control. 1997 Aug 8. 46(SS-4):1-15.
    National Center for Health Statistics: Utilization of short-stay hospitals:
    Annual summary for the United States.
    In: *Vital & Health Statistics*. Washington, DC. 1993. Series 13, number 128,
    Table 24. p42.

Chapter 2:   Morbidity and Mortality

3   A Standard Dictionary of the English Language. 20th Century Edition. 1907. s.v.
    "hyster-, hystero-."

4   Benrubi GI.
    History of hysterectomy.
    Jour Fla Med Assoc. 1988. 75(8):533-8

5   **National Center for Health Statistics: Utilization of short-stay hospitals:**
    Annual summary for the United States. 1975.
    In: *Vital & Health Statistics*. Washington, DC. Series 13, number 31. Table 23.
    p54.

6   **National Center for Health Statistics: Utilization of short-stay hospitals:**
    Annual summary for the United States.
    In: *Vital & Health Statistics*. Washington, DC. Series 13, number 128. Table 22.
    p 40.

7   Pokras R, Hufnagel VG.
    Hysterectomies in the United States, 1965-84: Data from the National Health
    Survey.
    In: *Vital & Health Statistics*. Washington, DC. CDC. Series 13, number 92.
    Lepine LA, Hillis SD, Marchbanks PA, et al.
    Hysterectomy surveillance—United States, 1980 -1993.
    MMWR, Center For Disease Control. 1997 Aug 8. 46(SS-4):1-15.
    National Center for Health Statistics: Utilization of short-stay hospitals:
    Annual summary for the United States.
    In: *Vital & Health Statistics*. Washington, DC. Series 13, number 128. Table 22.
    p 40.

8   Lepine LA, Hillis SD, Marchbanks PA, et al.
        Hysterectomy surveillance—United States, 1980 -1993.
        MMWR, Center For Disease Control. 1997 Aug 8. 46(SS-4):1-15.
        Luoto R, Kaprio J, Keskimaki I, Pohjanlahti J-P, Rutanen E-M.
        Incidence, causes and surgical methods for hysterectomy in Finland, 1987-1989.
        Inter Jour Epidemiol. 1994 Apr. 23(2):348-358.
        Gitsch G, Berger E, Tatra G.
        Trends in thirty years of vaginal hysterectomy.
        Surgery Gynecol Obstet. 1991 Mar. 172(3):207-210.
        Amirikia H, Evans TN.
        Ten-year review of hysterectomies: trends, indications, and risks.
        Amer Jour Obstet Gynecol. 1979 Jun. 134(4):431-7.

9   Boyd ME, Groome PA.
        The morbidity of abdominal hysterectomy.
        Canadian Jour Surg. 1993 Apr. 36(2):155-9.
        Chryssikopoulos A, Loghis C.
        Indications and results of total hysterectomy.
        Int Surg. 1986. 71:188-194.
        Wingo PA, Huezo CM, Rubin GL, et al.
        The mortality risk associated with hysterectomy.
        Amer Jour Obstet Gynecol. 1985 Aug 1. 152(7 pt 1): 803-8.

10   Easterday CL, Grimes DA, Riggs JA.
        Hysterectomy in the United States.
        Obstet Gynecol. 1983 Aug. 62(2):203-212.
        Amirikia H, Evans TN.
        Ten-year review of hysterectomies: trends, indications, and risks.
        Amer Jour Obstet Gynecol. 1979 Jun. 134(4):431-7.

11   Tindall VR.
        The national confidential enquiry into perioperative deaths.
        Brit Jour Obstet Gynaecol. 1994 June. 101:468-470.

12   Loft A, Andersen TF, Bronnum-Hansen H, Roepstorff C, Madsen M.
        Early postoperative mortality following hysterectomy. A Danish population based study, 1977-1981.
        Brit Jour Obstet Gynaecol. 1991 Feb. 98:147-154.

13   Lepine LA, Hillis SD, Marchbanks PA, et al.
        Hysterectomy surveillance—United States, 1980 -1993.
        MMWR, Center For Disease Control. 1997 Aug 8. 46(SS-4):1-15.

14   Boyd ME, Groome PA.
        The morbidity of abdominal hysterectomy.
        Canadian Jour Surg. 1993 Apr. 36(2):155-9.
        Dicker RC, Greenspan JR, Strauss LT, Cowart MR, et al.
        Complications of abdominal and vaginal hysterectomy among women of reproductive age in the United States: The Collaborative Review of Sterilization.
        Amer Jour Obstet Gynecol. 1982 Dec. 144(7):841-8.
        Senior CC, Steigrad SJ.
        Are preoperative antibiotics helpful in abdominal hysterectomy?
        Amer Jour Obstet Gynecol. 1986. 154:1004-8.
        Dwyer N, Hutton J, Stirrat GM.
        Randomised controlled trial comparing endometrial resection with abdominal hysterectomy for the surgical treatment of menorrhagia.

Brit Jour Obstet Gynaecol. 1993 Mar. 100:237-243.
Iverson RE, Chelmow D, et al.
Relative morbidity of abdominal hysterectomy and myomectomy for management of uterine leiomyomas.
Obstet Gynecol. 1996 Sept. 88(3):415-9.

15   Mittendorf R, Aronson MP, Berry RE, Williams MA, et al.
Avoiding serious infections associated with abdominal hysterectomy: a meta-analysis of antibiotic prophylaxis.
Amer Jour Obstet Gynecol. Nov 1993. 169(5) 1119-1124.
Dicker RC, Greenspan JR, Strauss LT, Cowart MR, et al.
Complications of abdominal and vaginal hysterectomy among women of reproductive age in the United States: The Collaborative Review of Sterilization.
Amer Jour Obstet Gynecol. 1982 Dec. 144(7):841-8.
Dwyer N, Hutton J, Stirrat GM.
Randomised controlled trial comparing endometrial resection with abdominal hysterectomy for the surgical treatment of menorrhagia.
Brit Jour Obstet Gynaecol. 1993 Mar. 100:237-243.
Senior CC, Steigrad SJ.
Are preoperative antibiotics helpful in abdominal hysterectomy?
Amer Jour Obstet Gynecol. 1986. 154:1004-8.

16   Prior A, Stanley KM, Smith ARB, Read NW.
Relation between hysterectomy and the irritable bowel: a prospective study.
Gut. 1992 Jun. 33(6):814-7.
Dicker RC, Greenspan JR, Strauss LT, Cowart MR, et al.
Complications of abdominal and vaginal hysterectomy among women of reproductive age in the United States: The Collaborative Review of Sterilization.
Amer Jour Obstet Gynecol. 1982 Dec. 144(7):841-8.
Kvist-Poulsen H, Borel J.
Iatrogenic femoral neuropathy subsequent to abdominal hysterectomy: incidence and prevention.
Obstet Gynecol. 1982 Oct. 60(4):516-520.
Boyd ME, Groome PA.
The morbidity of abdominal hysterectomy.
Canadian Jour Surg. 1993 Apr. 36(2):155-9.
Iverson RE, Chelmow D, et al.
Relative morbidity of abdominal hysterectomy and myomectomy for management of uterine leiomyomas.
Obstet Gynecol. 1996 Sept. 88(3):415-9.

17   Stricker B, Blanco J, Fox HE.
The gynecologic contribution to intestinal obstruction in females.
Jour Amer College Surg. 1994 June. 178(6):617-20.
Ratcliff JB, Kapernick P, Brooks GG, Dunnihoo DR.
Small bowel obstruction and previous gynecologic surgery.
South Med. Jour. 1983 Nov. 76(11):1349-1350.

18   Ratcliff JB, Kapernick P, Brooks GG, Dunnihoo DR.
Small bowel obstruction and previous gynecologic surgery.
South Med. Jour. 1983 Nov. 76(11):1349-1350.

19   Andersen TF, Loft A, et al.
Complications after hysterectomy: A Danish population based study 1978-1983.

Acta Obstet Gynecol Scand. 1993. 72:570-7.

20   Amirikia H, Evans TN.
        Ten-year review of hysterectomies: trends, indications, and risks.
        Amer Jour Obstet Gynecol. 1979 Jun. 134(4):431-7.
        Centerwall BS.
        Premenopausal hysterectomy and cardiovascular disease.
        Amer Jour Obstet Gynecol. 1981 Jan 1. 139(1):58-61.
        Richards DH.
        Depression after hysterectomy.
        Lancet. 1973 Aug 25. 2(7826):430-3.
        Hanley HG.
        The late urological complications of total hysterectomy.
        Brit Jour Urol. 1969. 41:682-4.
        Nathorst-Boos J, von Schoultz B.
        Psychological reactions and sexual life after hysterectomy with and without oophorectomy.
        Gynecol Obstet Invest. 1992. 34:97-101.

21   **Cancer facts & figures - 1996.**
        Atlanta, GA. American Cancer Society. 1996. Pub. 96-300M-No.5008.96:6.
        (Pamplet).

22   Oliver MF, Edin MD, Boyd GS.
        Effect of bilateral ovariectomy on coronary-artery disease and serum-lipid levels.
        Lancet. 1959 Oct. 2:690-4.
        Luoto R, Kaprio J, Reunanen A, Rutanen E-M.
        Cardiovascular morbidity in relation to ovarian function after hysterectomy.
        Obstet Gynecol. 1995 Apr. 85(4):515-522.
        Kannel WB, Hjortland MC, McNamara PM, Gordon T.
        Menopause and Risk of cardiovascular disease: The Framingham Study.
        Ann Internal Med. 1976 Oct. 85(4):447-452.
        Fast facts on osteoporosis.
        Washington, D.C. National Osteoporosis Foundation. 1998. (Internet)
        Galsworthy TD.
        The mechanism of an osteoporosis center.
        Orthopedic Clin North Amer. 1990 Jan. 21(1):163-9.
        Updated per author fax (1998 Mar 11).
        Deaths by leading cause: Deaths, by age and leading cause: 1994.
        In: *Statistical Abstract of the United States 1997.* 117th Ed. Washington, DC.
        Department of Commerce. Table no. 130 p 97.

23   Schofield MJ, Bennett A, Redman S, et al.
        Self-reported long-term outcomes of hysterectomy.
        Brit Jour Obstet Gynaecol. 1991 Nov. 98:1129-1136.

24   Gambone JC, Reiter RC, Lench JB.
        Short-term outcome of incidental hysterectomy at the time of adnexectomy for benign disease.
        Jour Women's Health. 1992. 1(3):197-200.

25   Gambone JC, Reiter RC, Lench JB.
        Short-term outcome of incidental hysterectomy at the time of adnexectomy for benign disease.
        Jour Women's Health. 1992. 1(3):197-200.

26   Opit LJ, Hobbs MST.
        Epidemics of procedures: growth in admissions to hospital in western Australia, 1972 to 1977.

Med Jour Aust. 1979 Oct 6. 2:378-380.

Pokras R, Hufnagel VG.
Hysterectomies in the United States, 1965-84: Data from the National Health Survey.
In: *Vital & Health Statistics.* Washington, DC. CDC. Series 13, number 92. pp1-31.

27   Lepine LA, Hillis SD, Marchbanks PA, et al.
Hysterectomy surveillance—United States, 1980 -1993.
MMWR, Center For Disease Control. 1997 Aug 8. 46(SS-4):1-15.

Luoto R, Kaprio J, Keskimaki I, Pohjanlahti J-P, Rutanen E-M.
Incidence, causes and surgical methods for hysterectomy in Finland, 1987-1989.
Inter Jour Epidemiol. 1994 Apr. 23(2):348-358.

28   Peng JJ.
30 years' experience of obstetric hysterectomy.
Chung-Hua Fu Chan Ko Tsa Chih Chinese Jour Obstet Gyn. 1991 Nov. 26(6):365-7 & 388-9. (Abstract).

Chan YG, Ho HK, Chen CY.
Abdominal hysterectomy: indications and complications.
Singapore Med Jour. 1993 Aug. 34(4): 337-40. (Abstract).

Chryssikopoulos A, Loghis C.
Indications and results of total hysterectomy.
Int Surg. 1986. 71:188-194.

Sahagun Quevedo JA, Perez Ruiz JC, Cherem B, Porras E.
Analysis of 1,000 hysterectomies. Technical simplifications and reflections. ISSSTE hospitals.
Ginecol Obstet de Mexico. 1994 Feb. 62:35-9. (Abstract).

Rizvi JH, Afzal W, Ali A, Khan K.
Was that hysterectomy really necessary? Audit of operative justification at the Aga Khan University Medical Center, Karachi.
Aust New Zeal Jour Obstet Gyn. 1991 Feb. 31(1):80-3.

29   Lepine LA, Hillis SD, Marchbanks PA, et al.
Hysterectomy surveillance—United States, 1980 -1993.
MMWR, Center For Disease Control. 1997 Aug 8. 46(SS-4):1-15.

30   Santow G, Bracher M.
Hysterectomy in Australia.
Aust. New Zealand Obstet Gynaecol. 1993 Feb. 33(1):105-6.

Dennerstein L, Shelley J, Smith AMA, Ryan M.
Hysterectomy experience among mid-aged Australian women.
Med Jour Aust. 1994 Sept 5. 161:311-3.

31   Vessey MP, Villard-Mackintosh L, McPherson K, Coulter A, Yeates D.
The epidemiology of hysterectomy: findings in a large cohort study.
Brit Jour Obstet Gynaecol. 1992 May. 99:402-7.

32   Luoto R, Kaprio J, Keskimaki I, Pohjanlahti J-P, Rutanen E-M.
Incidence, causes and surgical methods for hysterectomy in Finland, 1987-1989.
Inter Jour Epidemiol. 1994 Apr. 23(2):348-358.

33   Morley JE, Kaiser FE.
Sexual function with advancing age.
Med Clin North Amer. 1989 Nov. 73(6):1483-1495.

34   Parazzini F, Gastaldi A, Minini G, Centonze M, et al.
Prophylactic oophorectomy during hysterectomy for benign conditions.

Lancet. 1993 Apr 3. 341(8849):898-9. (Letter).
Indications, surgical modality and complications of hysterectomy for benign pathology: results of a Lombard study.
Ann Ostet Ginecol Med Perinat. 1993 May-Jun. 113(3):161-9. (Abstract).

35   Rizvi JH, Afzal W, Ali A, Khan K.
Was that hysterectomy really necessary? Audit of operative justification at the Aga Khan University Medical Center, Karachi.
Aust New Zeal Jour Obstet Gyn. 1991 Feb. 31(1):80-3.

36   Wongsa P.
Elective hysterectomy—trends at Angthong hospital.
Jour Med Assoc Thail. 1994 Jul. 77(7):384-7. (Abstract).

Chapter 3:   The Ovaries

37   Sightler SE, Boike GM, Estape RE, Averette HE.
Ovarian cancer in women with prior hysterectomy: a 14-year experience at the University of Miami.
Obstet Gynecol. 1991 Oct. 78(4):681-684.

Christ JE, Lotze EC.
The residual ovary syndrome.
Obstet Gynecol. 1975 Nov. 46(5):551-6.

Greenwald EF.
Ovarian Tumors.
Clin Obstet Gynecol. 1975 Dec. 18(4):61-86.

38   Lepine LA, Hillis SD, Marchbanks PA, et al.
Hysterectomy surveillance—United States, 1980 -1993.
MMWR, Center For Disease Control. 1997 Aug 8. 46(SS-4):1-15.

39   Adashi EY.
The climacteric ovary: A viable endocrine organ.
Semin Reprod Endocrinol. 1991 Aug. 9(3):200-5.

40   Longcope C, Hunter R, Franz C.
Steroid secretion by the postmenopausal ovary.
Amer Jour Obstet Gynecol. 1980 Nov 1. 138(5):564-8.

Kobayashi M, Nakano R, Shima K.
Immunohistochemical localization of pituitary gonadotropins and estrogen in human postmenopausal ovaries.
Acta Obstet Gynecol Scand. 1993. 72:76-80.

41   Adashi EY.
The climacteric ovary: A viable endocrine organ.
Semin Reprod Endocrinol. 1991 Aug. 9(3):200-5.

42   Adashi EY.
The climacteric ovary: A viable endocrine organ.
Semin Reprod Endocrinol. 1991 Aug. 9(3):200-5.

43   Sluijmer AV, Heineman MJ, De Jong FH, Evers JLH.
Endocrine activity of the postmenopausal ovary: the effects of pituitary down-regulation and oophorectomy.
Jour Clin Endocrin Metab. 1995 Jul. 80(7):2163-7.

Botella-Llusia J, Oriol-Bosch A, Sanchez-Garrido F, et al.
Testosterone and 17β-oestradiol Secretion of the human ovary. II. Normal postmenopausal women, postmenopausal women with endometrial hyperplasia and postmenopausal women with adenocarcinoma of the endometrium.

Maturitas. 1979. 2:7-12.

44   Hollenbeck ZJR.
Ovarian cancer-prophylactic oophorectomy.
Amer Surg. 1955. 21:442-6.

45   Aitken JM, Hart DM, Lindsay R.
Oestrogen replacement therapy for prevention of osteoporosis after oophorectomy.
Brit Med Jour. 1973 Sep 8. 3:515-518.

Urban RJ, Bodenburg YH, Gilkison C, Foxworth J, et al.
Testosterone administration to elderly men increases skeletal muscle strength and protein synthesis.
Amer Jour Physiol. 1995 Nov. 269(5 Pt 1):E820-6.

Maheux R, Naud F, Rioux M, Grenier R, Lemay A, et al.
A randomized, double-blind, placebo-controlled study on the effect of conjugated estrogens on skin thickness.
Amer Jour Obstet Gynecol. 1994 Feb. 170(2):642-9.

46   Oliver MF, Edin MD, Boyd GS.
Effect of bilateral ovariectomy on coronary-artery disease and serum-lipid levels.
Lancet. 1959 Oct. 2:690-4.

Wuest JH, Dry TJ, Edwards JE.
The degree of coronary atherosclerosis in bilaterally oophorectomized women.
Circulation. 1953 June. 7(6):801-9.

De Leo V, Lanzetta D, D D'Antona, Danero S.
Growth hormone secretion in premenopausal women before and after ovariectomy: effect of hormone replacement therapy.
Fertil Steril. 1993 Aug. 60(2):268-271.

Salomon F, Cuneo RC, Hesp R, Sonksen PH.
The effects of treatment with recombinant human growth hormone on body composition and metabolism in adults with growth hormone deficiency.
New Engl Jour Med. 1989 Dec 28. 321(26):1797-1803.

47   Luoto R, Kaprio J, Reunanen A, Rutanen E-M.
Cardiovascular morbidity in relation to ovarian function after hysterectomy.
Obstet Gynecol. 1995 Apr. 85(4):515-522.

48   Sherwin BB, Gelfand MM.
Differential symptom response to parenteral estrogen and/or androgen administration in the surgical menopause. Transactions of the 14th annual meeting of the society of obstetricians and gynaecologists of Canada.
Amer Jour Obstet Gynecol. 1985 Jan 15. 151(2):153-160.

Genazzani AR, Facchinetti F, Ricci-Danero MG, Parrini D, et al.
Beta-lipotropin and beta-endorphin in physiological and surgical menopause.
Jour Endocrinol Invest. 1981 Oct. 4(4):375-8.

49   Kilkku P, Gronroos M, Hirvonen T, Rauramo L.
Supravaginal uterine amputation vs. hysterectomy: effects on libido and orgasm.
Acta Obstet Gynecol Scand. 1983. 62:147-152.

50   Khan-Dawood FS.
Human corpus luteum: immunocytochemical localization of epidermal growth factor.
Fertil Steril. 1987 June. 47(6):916-9.

Pepperell JR, Nemeth G, Roa L, Yamada Y, Palumbo A, et al.
Intraovarian regulation by the ovarian renin-angiotensin system.

Aust New Zealand Obstet Gynaecol. 1994. 34(3):288-292.

Vermeulen A.

Sex hormone status of the postmenopausal woman.

Maturitas. 1980 Jul 1. 2(2):81-9.

51   Hollenbeck ZJR.

Ovarian cancer-prophylactic oophorectomy.

Amer Surg. 1955. 21:442-6.

52   Annegers JF, Strom H, Decker DG, Dockerty MB, O'Fallon M.

Ovarian cancer: incidence and case-control study.

Cancer. 1979. 43:723-729.

Loft A, Lidegaard O, Tabor A.

Incidence of ovarian cancer after hysterectomy: a nationwide controlled follow up.

Brit Jour Obstet Gynaecol. 1997 Nov. 104:1296-1301.

Hartge P, Hoover R, et al.

Menopause and ovarian cancer.

Amer Jour Epidemiol. 1988 May. 127(5):990-8.

Hankinson SE, Hunter DJ, Colditz GA, Willett WC, Stampfer MJ, et al.

Tubal ligation, hysterectomy, and risk of ovarian cancer: a prospective study.

Jour Amer Med Assoc. 1993 Dec 15. 270(23):2813-8.

53   Parazzini F, Negri E, La Vecchia C, Luchini L, Mezzopane R.

Hysterectomy, oophorectomy, and subsequent ovarian cancer risk.

Obstet Gynecol. 1993 Mar. 81(3)363-6.

54   Hartge P, Whittemore AS, Itnyre J, et al.

Rates and risks of ovarian cancer in subgroups of white women in the United States.

Obstet Gynecol. 1994 Nov. 84(5):760-4.

55   Weiss NS, Harlow BL.

Why does hysterectomy without bilateral oophorectomy influence the subsequent incidence of ovarian cancer?

Amer Jour Epidemiol. 1986 Nov. 124(5):856-8.

Green A, Purdie D, Bain C, et al.

Tubal sterilisation, hysterectomy and decreased risk of ovarian cancer.

Int Jour Cancer. 1997. 71:948-951.

56   Garcia C, Cutler WB.

Preservation of the ovary: a reevaluation.

Fert Steril. 1984 Oct. 42(4):510-4.

57   Rudy DR, Bush IM.

Hysterectomy and sexual dysfunction: you can help.

Patient Care. 1992 Sept 30. 26(15):67-82.

58   Hollenbeck ZJR.

Ovarian cancer-prophylactic oophorectomy.

Amer Surg. 1955. 21:442-6.

Hagstad A, Janson PO.

The epidemiology of climacteric symptoms.

Acta Obstet Gynecol Scand Suppl. 1986. 134:59-65.

59   Hreshchyshyn MM, Hopkins A, et al.

Effects of natural menopause, hysterectomy, and oophorectomy on lumbar spine and femoral neck bone densities.

Obstet Gynecol. 1988 Oct. 72(4):631-8.

Parrish HM, Carr CA, Hall DG, King TM.

Time interval from castration in premenopausal women to development of excessive coronary atherosclerosis.

Amer Jour Obstet Gynecol. 1967 Sept 15. 99(2):155-162.

60   Garcia C, Cutler WB.
        Preservation of the ovary: a reevaluation.
        Fert Steril. 1984 Oct. 42(4):510-4.

61   Siddle N, Sarrel P, Whitehead M.
        **The effect of hysterectomy on the age at ovarian failure: identification of a
        subgroup of women with premature loss of ovarian function and literature
        review.**
        Fertil Steril. 1987 Jan. 47(1):94-100.

        Parker M, Bosscher J, Barnhill D, Park R.
        **Ovarian management during radical hysterectomy in the premenopausal
        patient.**
        Obstet Gynecol. 1993 Aug. 82(2):187-190.

62   Parker M, Bosscher J, Barnhill D, Park R.
        **Ovarian management during radical hysterectomy in the premenopausal
        patient.**
        Obstet Gynecol. 1993 Aug. 82(2):187-190.

63   Parker M, Bosscher J, Barnhill D, Park R.
        **Ovarian management during radical hysterectomy in the premenopausal
        patient.**
        Obstet Gynecol. 1993 Aug. 82(2):187-190.

64   Plockinger B, Kolbl H.
        **Development of ovarian pathology after hysterectomy without oophorec-
        tomy.**
        Jour Amer College Surg. 1994 Jun. 178(6):581-5.

        Parker M, Bosscher J, Barnhill D, Park R.
        **Ovarian management during radical hysterectomy in the premenopausal
        patient.**
        Obstet Gynecol. 1993 Aug. 82(2):187-190.

65   Seeley T.
        Oestrogen replacement therapy after hysterectomy.
        Brit Med Jour. 1992 Oct 3. 305(6857):811-2.

66   Watson, NR, Studd JWW, Garnett T, Savvas M, Milligan P.
        Bone loss after hysterectomy with ovarian conservation.
        Obstet Gynecol. 1995 Jul. 86(1):72-7.

67   Vuorento T, Maenpaa J, Huhtaniemi I.
        **Follow-up of ovarian endocrine function in premenopausal women after
        hysterectomy by daily measurements of salivary progesterone.**
        Clin Endocrinol. 1992 May. 36(5):505-510.

68   Oldenhave A, Jaszmann LJB, Everaerd W, Haspels AA.
        **Hysterectomized women with ovarian conservation report more severe
        climacteric complaints than do normal climacteric women of similar age.**
        Amer Jour Obstet Gynecol. 1993 Mar. 168(3 pt 1):765-771.

        Hreshchyshyn MM, Hopkins A, et al.
        **Effects of natural menopause, hysterectomy, and oophorectomy on lumbar
        spine and femoral neck bone densities.**
        Obstet Gynecol. 1988 Oct. 72(4):631-8.

        Centerwall BS.
        Premenopausal hysterectomy and cardiovascular disease.
        Amer Jour Obstet Gynecol. 1981 Jan 1. 139(1):58-61.

        Spector TD, Brown GC, Silman AJ.
        **Increased rates of previous hysterectomy and gynaecological operations in
        women with osteoarthritis.**

BMJ. 1988 Oct 8. 297:899-900.

Nathorst-Boos J, von Schoultz B.

Psychological reactions and sexual life after hysterectomy with and without oophorectomy.

Gynecol Obstet Invest. 1992. 34:97-101.

69   Bukovsky I, Halperin R, Schneider D, Golan A, Hertzianu I, Herman A.

Ovarian function following abdominal hysterectomy with and without unilateral oophorectomy.

Europ Jour Obstet Gynecol Repro Biol. 1995 Jan. 58(1):29-32.

70   Luoto R, Kaprio J, Reunanen A, Rutanen E-M.

Cardiovascular morbidity in relation to ovarian function after hysterectomy.

Obstet Gynecol. 1995 Apr. 85(4):515-522.

Siddle N, Sarrel P, Whitehead M.

The effect of hysterectomy on the age at ovarian failure: identification of a subgroup of women with premature loss of ovarian function and literature review.

Fertil Steril. 1987 Jan. 47(1):94-100.

71   Kaiser R, Kusche M, Wurz H.

Hormone levels in women after hysterectomy.

Arch Gynecol Obstet. 1989. 244:169-173.

72   Sessums JV, Murphy DP.

Hysterectomy and the artificial menopause: review of literature, report of ninety-one cases.

Surg Gynecol Obstet. 1932 Jan-Mar. 54:286-9.

73   Siddle N, Sarrel P, Whitehead M.

The effect of hysterectomy on the age at ovarian failure: identification of a subgroup of women with premature loss of ovarian function and literature review.

Fertil Steril. 1987 Jan. 47(1):94-100.

Gambrell RD.

The menopause: benefits and risks of estrogen-progestogen replacement therapy.

Fertil Steril. 1982 Apr. 37(4):457-474.

74   Sessums JV, Murphy DP.

Hysterectomy and the artificial menopause: review of literature, report of ninety-one cases.

Surg Gynecol Obstet. 1932 Jan-Mar. 54:286-9.

Kretzschmar NR, Gardiner S.

A consideration of the surgical menopause after hysterectomy and the occurrence of cancer in the stump following subtotal hysterectomy.

Amer Jour Obstet Gynecol. 1935. 29:168-175.

75   Siddle N, Sarrel P, Whitehead M.

The effect of hysterectomy on the age at ovarian failure: identification of a subgroup of women with premature loss of ovarian function and literature review.

Fertil Steril. 1987 Jan. 47(1):94-100.

Erman A, Chen-Gal B, van Dijk DJ, Sulkes J, Kaplan B, et al.

Ovarian angiotensin-converting enzyme activity in humans: relationship to estradiol, age, and uterine pathology.

Jour Clin Endocrinol Metab. 1996. 81(3):1104-7.

76   DeStefano F, Perlman JA, Peterson HB, et al.

Long-term risk of menstrual disturbances after tubal sterilization.

Amer Jour Obstet Gynecol. 1985 Aug 1. 152(7Pt1):835-841.
Radwanska E, Headley SK, Dmowski P.
Evaluation of ovarian function after tubal sterilization.
Jour Reprod Med. 1982 July. 27(7):376-384.

77   Dippel AL.
The role of hysterectomy in the production of menopausal symptoms.
Amer Jour Obstet Gynecol. 1939. 37:111-3.

78   Janson PO, Jansson I.
The acute effect of hysterectomy on ovarian blood flow.
Amer Jour Obstet Gynecol. 1977 Feb. 127(4):349-352.

79   Borell U. Fernstrom I.
The adnexal branches of the uterine artery - An arteriographic study in human subjects.
Acta Radiol. 1953 Jul. 40:561-582.

80   Vermeulen A.
Sex hormone status of the postmenopausal woman.
Maturitas. 1980 Jul 1. 2(2):81-9.

81   Lindhard A, Nilas L.
The postmenopausal ovary—should it be preserved?
Ugeskrift for Laeger. 1994 Nov 21. 156(47):7018-7023. (Abstract).

82   Pepperell JR, Nemeth G, Roa L, Yamada Y, Palumbo A, et al.
Intraovarian regulation by the ovarian renin-angiotensin system.
Aust New Zealand Obstet Gynaecol. 1994. 34(3):288-292.

Chapter 4:   The Cervix IS Important

83   Grimes DA.
Shifting indications for hysterectomy: nature, nurture, or neither?
Lancet. 1994 Dec 17. 344(8938):1652-3.

84   Rudy DR, Bush IM.
Hysterectomy and sexual dysfunction: you can help.
Patient Care. 1992 Sept 30. 26(15):67-82.

85   Edvardsen L, Madsen EM.
Supravaginal or total hysterectomy?
Ugeskrift For Laeger. 1994 Aug 15. 156(33):4694-9. (Abstract).

86   Blakiston's Pocket Medical Dictionary. 3rd Ed., s.v. "hysterectomy."

87   **What you need to know about cancer of the uterus.**
Bethesda, MD. National Cancer Institute. 1988 Aug. 1C(25). (Pamphlet).

88   **Hysterectomy prevalence and death rates for cervical cancer—United States, 1965-1988.**
MMWR. U.S. CDC. 1992 Jan 17. 41(2): 17-21.
Epidemiological and vital statisitics report.
World Health Organization. 1964. 17:700.

89   Pokras R, Hufnagel VG.
Hysterectomies in the United States, 1965-84: Data from the National Health Survey.
In: *Vital & Health Statistics.* Washington, DC. CDC. Series 13, number 92. pp1-31.

90   **Hysterectomy prevalence and death rates for cervical cancer—United States, 1965-1988.**
MMWR. U.S. CDC. 1992 Jan 17. 41(2): 17-21.
Cancer rates and risks.
US Dept of Health and Human Services, Public Health Service, National

Institutes of Health. 1996. (Pamphlet).

91 Boyd ME, Groome PA.
The morbidity of abdominal hysterectomy.
Canadian Jour Surg. 1993 Apr. 36(2):155-9.
Chryssikopoulos A, Loghis C.
Indications and results of total hysterectomy.
Int Surg. 1986. 71:188-194.
Wingo PA, Huezo CM, Rubin GL, et al.
The mortality risk associated with hysterectomy.
Amer Jour Obstet Gynecol. 1985 Aug 1. 152(7 pt 1): 803-8.

92 **Hysterectomy prevalence and death rates for cervical cancer—United States, 1965-1988.**
MMWR. U.S. CDC. 1992 Jan 17. 41(2): 17-21.

93 Kretzschmar NR, Gardiner S.
A consideration of the surgical menopause after hysterectomy and the occurrence of cancer in the stump following subtotal hysterectomy.
Amer Jour Obstet Gynecol. 1935. 29:168-175.

94 Wright RC.
Hysterectomy: past, present, and future.
Obstet Gynecol. 1969 Apr. 33(4):560-3.

95 Kilkku P, Gronroos M.
Peroperative electrocoagulation of endocervical mucosa and later carcinoma of the cervical stump.
Acta Obstet Gynecol Scand. 1982. 61:265-7.

96 Benrubi GI.
History of hysterectomy.
Jour Fla Med Assoc. 1988. 75(8):533-8.

97 Sahagun Quevedo JA, Perez Ruiz JC, Cherem B, Porras E.
Analysis of 1,000 hysterectomies. Technical simplifications and reflections. ISSSTE hospitals.
Ginecol Obstet de Mexico. 1994 Feb. 62:35-9. (Abstract).

98 Nathorst-Boos J, Fuchs T, von Schoultz B.
Consumer's attitude to hysterectomy: the experience of 678 women.
Acta Obstet Gynecol Scand. 1992. 71:230-4.
Peng JJ.
30 years' experience of obstetric hysterectomy.
Chung-Hua Fu Chan Ko Tsa Chih Chinese Jour Obstet Gyn. 1991 Nov. 26(6):365-7 & 388-9. (Abstract).

99 Vara P, Kinnunen O.
Total versus subtotal abdominal hysterectomy.
Acta Obstet Gynecol Scand. 1953. 31(suppl 5):5-43.

100 Soper DE.
Upper genital tract infections.
In: *Textbook of Gynecology.* ed by Copeland LJ, Jarrell JF, McGregor JA. Philadelphia, PA. W.B. Saunders Co. 1993 p517.

101 Charbonnel B, Kremer M, Gerozissis K, Dray F.
Human cervical mucus contains large amounts of prostaglandins.
Fertil Steril. 1982 Jul. 38(1):109-111.
Vander AJ, Sherman JH, Luciano DS.
The internal environment and homeostasis.
In: *Human Physiology: The Mechanisms of Body Function.* 2nd ed. McGraw-

Hill. 1975. Ch. 5. pp129-130.

Duboff GS, Penner JA, Rohwedder J.
Effect of prostaglandins E1, E2 and F2a on human blood coagulation.
Nature. 1974 Oct 4. 251:430-1.

Dray F, Charbonnel B, Maclouf J.
Radioimmunoassay of prostaglandins Fa, E1 and E2 in human plasma.
Eur Jour Clin Invest. 1975. 5:311-8.

102   Charbonnel B, Kremer M, Gerozissis K, Dray F.
Human cervical mucus contains large amounts of prostaglandins.
Fertil Steril. 1982 Jul. 38(1):109-111.

103   Yuen PM, Rogers MS.
Laparoscopic hysterectomy: do we need to remove the cervix?
Aust New Zealand Jour Obstet Gynaecol. 1994. 34(4):464-6.

Weingold AB.
Gross and microscopic anatomy.
In: *Principles and Practice of Clinical Gynecology.* ed. by Kase NB, Weingold AB, Gershenson DM. 2nd ed. Edinburgh, England. Churchill Livingstone Inc. 1990. Ch. 1. p26.

Wood C, Maher P, Hill D, Selwood T.
Hysterectomy: a time of change.
Med Jour Aust. 1992 Nov 16. 157:651-3.

104   Herbst AL, et al.
Disorders of abdominal wall and pelvic support.
In: *Comprehensive Gynecology.* ed. by Manning S. St. Louis, MI. Mosby-Year Book, Inc. 1992. Ch. 19. p594.

105   Weingold AB.
Gross and microscopic anatomy.
In: *Principles and Practice of Clinical Gynecology.* ed. by Kase NB, Weingold AB, Gershenson DM. 2nd ed. Edinburgh, England. Churchill Livingstone Inc. 1990. Ch. 1. p26.

106   Kilkku P, Hirvonen T, Gronroos M.
Supra-vaginal uterine amputation vs. abdominal hysterectomy: the effects on urinary symptoms with special reference to pollakisuria, nocturia, dysuria.
Maturitas. 1981 Dec. 3(3-4):197-204.

107   Vervest HA, deJonge MK, Vervest T, et al.
Micturition symptoms and urinary incontinence after non-radical hysterectomy.
Acta Obstet Gynecol Scand. 1988. 67:141-146.

Smith AN, Varma JS, et al.
Disordered colorectal motility in intractable constipation following hysterectomy.
Brit Jour Surg. 1990 Dec. 77:1361-6.

108   Kilkku P, Gronroos M, Hirvonen T, Rauramo L.
Supravaginal uterine amputation vs. hysterectomy: effects on libido and orgasm.
Acta Obstet Gynecol Scand. 1983. 62:147-152.

109   Herbst AL, et al.
Anatomy.
In: *Comprehensive Gynecology.* ed. by Manning S. St. Louis, MI. Mosby-Year Book, Inc. 1992. Ch. 3. p52.

Kinsey AC, et al.
Anatomy of sexual response and orgasm.
In: *Sexual behavior in the human female.* 1953.

Philadelphia, PA. W.B. Saunders Co. 1953. p577.

Clark L.

Is there a difference between a clitoral and a vaginal orgasm?
Jour Sex Research. 1970 Feb. 6(1):25-8.

Zussman L, Zussman S, Sunley R, Bjornson E.

Sexual response after hysterectomy-oophorectomy: recent studies and reconsideration of psychogenesis.
Amer Jour Obstet Gynecol. 1981 Aug 1. 140(7):725-9.

110   Hasson HM.

Cervical removal at hysterectomy for benign disease: risks and benefits.
Jour Reprod Med. 1993 Oct. 38(10):781-790.

111   Filiberti A, Regazzoni M, Garavoglia M, Perilli C, Alpinelli P, et al.

Problems after hysterectomy. A comparative content analysis of 60 interviews with cancer and non-cancer hysterectomized women.
Eur Jour Gynaec Oncol. 1991. XII(6):445-9.

Kilkku P, Gronroos M, Hirvonen T, Rauramo L.

Supravaginal uterine amputation vs. hysterectomy: effects on libido and orgasm.
Acta Obstet Gynecol Scand. 1983. 62:147-152.

Nathorst-Boos J, von Schoultz B.

Psychological reactions and sexual life after hysterectomy with and without oophorectomy.
Gynecol Obstet Invest. 1992. 34:97-101.

Raboch J, Boudnik V, Raboch J Jr.

Sex life following hysterectomy.
Geburtshilfe Frauenheilkd. 1985 Jan. 45(1):48-50. (Abstract).

112   Edvardsen L, Madsen EM.

Supravaginal or total hysterectomy?
Ugeskrift for Laeger. 1994 Aug 15. 156(33):4694-9. (Abstract).

113   Kilkku P, Gronroos M, Hirvonen T, Rauramo L.

Supravaginal uterine amputation vs. hysterectomy: effects on libido and orgasm.
Acta Obstet Gynecol Scand. 1983. 62:147-152.

114   Kinsey AC, et al.

Anatomy of sexual response and orgasm.
In: *Sexual behavior in the human female.* 1953.
Philadelphia, PA. W.B. Saunders Co. 1953. pp577,584.

115   Hasson HM.

Cervical removal at hysterectomy for benign disease: risks and benefits.
Jour Reprod Med. 1993 Oct. 38(10):781-790.

Chapter 5:   High Blood Pressure

116   Centerwall BS.

Premenopausal hysterectomy and cardiovascular disease.
Amer Jour Obstet Gynecol. 1981 Jan 1. 139(1):58-61.

Punnonen R, Ikalainen M, Seppala E.

Premenopausal hysterectomy and risk of cardiovascular disease.
Lancet. 1987 May 16. 1(8542):1139.

Kannel WB, Hjortland MC, McNamara PM, Gordon T.

Menopause and Risk of cardiovascular disease: The Framingham Study.

Ann Internal Med. 1976 Oct. 85(4):447-452.

117 **About high blood pressure.**
Dallas, TX. American Heart Association. Fighting heart disease and stroke. 1993. 50-1055. (Pamphlet).

118 Luoto R, Kaprio J, Reunanen A, Rutanen E-M.
Cardiovascular morbidity in relation to ovarian function after hysterectomy.
Obstet Gynecol. 1995 Apr. 85(4):515-522.

119 Luoto R, Kaprio J, Reunanen A, Rutanen E-M.
Cardiovascular morbidity in relation to ovarian function after hysterectomy.
Obstet Gynecol. 1995 Apr. 85(4):515-522.

120 **The fifth report of the Joint National Committee on detection, evaluation, and treatment of high blood pressure (JNC V). Special Article.**
Arch Intern Med. 1993 Jan 25. 153:154-183.

121 Stokes JS III, Kannel WB, et al.
The relative importance of selected risk factors for various manifestations of cardiovascular disease among men and women from 35 to 64 years old: 30 years of follow-up in the Framinghan Study.
Circulation. 1987 Jun. 75(suppl V):V65-V73.

122 Williams GH, Moore TJ.
Hormonal aspects of hypertension.
In: *Endocrinology.* ed. by DeGroot LJ, et al. 3rd ed. Philadelphia, PA. WB Saunders Co. 1995. Vol. 3. Ch. 155. pp2917-2920.

Vander AJ, Sherman JH, Luciano DS.
Regulation of water and electrolyte balance.
In: *Human Physiology: The Mechanisms of Body Function.* 2nd ed. McGraw-Hill. 1975. Ch. 11. pp336-7.

123 Sealey JE, Glorioso N, Itskovitz J, et al.
Plasma prorenin during early pregnancy: ovarian secretion under gonadotropin control?
Jour Hypertension. 1986. 4(Suppl 5):S92-S95.

Woods LL.
Role of angiotensin II and prostaglandins in the regulation of uteroplacental blood flow.
Amer Jour Physiol. 1993 Mar. 264(3Pt2):R584-90.

Palumbo A, Jones C, Lightman A, Carcangiu ML, et al.
Immunohistochemical localization of the renin and angiotensin II in human ovaries.
Amer Jour Obstet Gynecol. 1989 Jan. 160(1):8-14.

Lightman A, Palumbo A, DeCherney AH, Naftolin F.
The ovarian renin-angiotensin system.
Semin Repro Endocrinol. 1989 Feb. 7(1):79-87.

Pepperell JR, Yamada Y, Nemeth G, Palumbo A, et al.
The ovarian renin-angiotensin system. A paracrine-intracrine regulator of ovarian function.
Adv Exper Med Biol. 1995. 377:379-389.

van Sande ME, Scharpe SL, Neels HM, Van Camp KO.
Distribution of angiotensin converting enzyme in human tissues.
Clinica Chimica Acta. 1985. 147:255-260.

Pepperell JR, Nemeth G, Roa L, Yamada Y, Palumbo A, et al.
Intraovarian regulation by the ovarian renin-angiotensin system.
Aust New Zealand Obstet Gynaecol. 1994. 34(3):288-292.

Erman A, Chen-Gal B, van Dijk DJ, Sulkes J, Kaplan B, et al.
Ovarian angiotensin-converting enzyme activity in humans: relationship to estradiol, age, and uterine pathology.

Jour Clin Endocrinol Metab. 1996. 81(3):1104-7.

Yoshimura Y.

The ovarian renin-angiotensin system in reproductive physiology.

Frontiers Neuroend. 1997. 18:247-291.

124   Wilson M, Morganti AA, Zervoudakis I, et al.

Blood pressure, the renin-aldosterone system and sex steroids throughout normal pregnancy.

Amer Jour Med. 1980 Jan. 68:97-104.

Leckie BJ, McConnell A, Grant J, et al.

An inactive renin in human plasma.

Circ Res. 1977 May. 40(5)(S1):I46-I51.

125   Palumbo A, Jones C, Lightman A, Carcangiu ML, et al.

Immunohistochemical localization of the renin and angiotensin II in human ovaries.

Amer Jour Obstet Gynecol. 1989 Jan. 160(1):8-14.

Derkx FHM, Alberda AT, De Jong FH, et al.

Source of plasma prorenin in early and late pregnancy: observations in patient with primary ovarian failure.

Jour Clin Endocrinol Metab. 1987. 65:349-354.

Leckie BJ, McConnell A, Grant J, et al.

An inactive renin in human plasma.

Circ Res. 1977 May. 40(5)(S1):I46-I51.

Sealey JE, Glorioso N, Itskovitz J, et al.

Plasma prorenin during early pregnancy: ovarian secretion under gonadotropin control?

Jour Hypertension. 1986. 4(Suppl 5):S92-S95.

126   Alderman MH, Madhavan S, Cohen H, Sealey JE, Laragh JH.

Low urinary sodium is associated with greater risk of myocardial infarction among treated hypertensive men.

Hypertension. 1995 June. 25(6):1144-1152.

127   Sealey JE, Moon C, Laragh JH, Atlas SA.

Plasma prorenin in normal, hypertensive, and anephric subjects and its effect on renin measurements.

Circ Res. 1977 May. (Suppl I) 40(5):I41-I45.

128   Williams GH, Moore TJ.

Hormonal aspects of hypertension.

In: *Endocrinology.* ed. by DeGroot LJ, et al. 3rd ed. Philadelphia, PA. WB Saunders Co. 1995. Vol. 3. Ch. 155. pp2917-2920.

129   Alderman MH, Madhavan S, Cohen H, Sealey JE, Laragh JH.

Low urinary sodium is associated with greater risk of myocardial infarction among treated hypertensive men.

Hypertension. 1995 June. 25(6):1144-1152.

130   Wilding JP, Ghatei MA, Bloom SR.

Hormones of the gastrointestinal tract.

In: *Endocrinology.* ed. by DeGroot LJ, et al. 3rd ed. Philadelphia, PA. WB Saunders Co. 1995. Vol. 3. Ch. 153. p2881.

Kohlmann O Jr., Cesaretti ML, et al.

Role of Substance P in blood pressure regulation in salt-dependent experimental hypertension.

Hypertension. 1997. 29(part 2):506-9.

131   Duval P, Lenoir V, et al.

Substance P and neurokinin A variations throughout the rat estrous cycle; comparison with ovariectomized and male rats: I. plasma, hypothalamus, anterior and posterior pituitary.

Jour Neurosci Research. 1996. 45:598-609.

132   Tagawa H, Shimokawa H, Tagawa T, et al.
        **Short-term estrogen augments both nitric oxide-mediated and non-nitric
        oxide-mediated endothelium-dependent forearm vasodilation in postmeno-
        pausal women.**
        Jour Cardiovasc Pharmacol. 1997. 30(4):481-8.

133   Tagawa H, Shimokawa H, Tagawa T, et al.
        **Short-term estrogen augments both nitric oxide-mediated and non-nitric
        oxide-mediated endothelium-dependent forearm vasodilation in postmeno-
        pausal women.**
        Jour Cardiovasc Pharmacol. 1997. 30(4):481-8.

134   Amstein R, Fetkovska N, Buhler FR.
        **Age, platelet serotonin kinetics and 5HT2-receptor blockade in essential
        hypertension.**
        Jour Human Hypertension. 1990. 4:441-4.
        Guicheney P, Devynck M, et al.
        **Platelet 5-HT content and uptake in essential hypertension: role of endog-
        enous digitalis-like factors and plasma cholesterol.**
        Jour Hypertension. 1988. 6(11):873-9.

135   Gujrati VR, Goyal A, et al.
        **Relevance of platelet serotonergic mechanisms in pregnancy induced
        hypertension.**
        Life Sci. 1994. 55(4):327-335.

136   Kimura T, Yoshida Y, Toda N.
        **Mechanisms of relaxation induced by prostaglandins in isolated canine
        uterine arteries.**
        Amer Jour Obstet Gynecol. 1992 Nov. 167(5):1409-1416.
        Shelton JD.
        Prostacyclin from the uterus and woman's cardiovascular advantage.
        Prostaglandins Leukotrienes Med. 1982. 8:459-466.
        Moncada S, Vane JR.
        **Arachidonic acid metabolites and the interactions between platelets and
        blood-vessel walls.**
        New Eng Jour Med. 1979 May 17. 300(20):1142-7.

137   Moncada S, Vane JR.
        **Arachidonic acid metabolites and the interactions between platelets and
        blood-vessel walls.**
        New Eng Jour Med. 1979 May 17. 300(20):1142-7.
        Kimura T, Okamura T, Yoshida Y, Toda N.
        **Relaxant responses to prostaglandin F2a and E2 of isolated human uterine
        arteries.**
        Jour Cariovascul Pharmacol. 1995 Aug. 26(2):333-8.
        Schramm W, Einer-Jensen N, Brown MB, Mc Cracken JA.
        **Effect of four primary prostaglandins and relaxin on blood flow in the ovine
        endometrium and myometrium.**
        Biol. Reprod. 1984. 30:523-531.
        Clark KE, Austin JE, Stys SJ.
        **Effect of bisenoic prostaglandins on the uterine vasculature of the nonpreg-
        nant sheep.**
        Prostaglandins. 1981 Sept. 22(3):333-348.

138   Vander AJ, Sherman JH, Luciano DS.
        Respiration.
        In: *Human Physiology: The Mechanisms of Body Function.* 2nd ed. McGraw-

Hill. 1975. Ch. 10. pp283-318.

Linman JW.
Polycythemia (Erythrocytosis).
In: *Principles of Hematology*. New York, NY. The Macmillan Co. 1966. Ch. 6.
pp295-7.

Linman JW.
The blood cells (general considerations).
In: *Principles of Hematology*. New York, NY. The Macmillan Co. 1966. Ch. 1.
p12 p21.

139   Vander AJ, Sherman JH, Luciano DS.
Respiration.
In: *Human Physiology: The Mechanisms of Body Function*. 2nd ed. McGraw-
Hill. 1975. Ch. 10. p314.

Linman JW.
Polycythemia (Erythrocytosis).
In: *Principles of Hematology*. New York, NY. The Macmillan Co. 1966. Ch. 6.
pp295.

140   Shelton JD.
Prostacyclin from the uterus and woman's cardiovascular advantage.
Prostaglandins Leukotrienes Med. 1982. 8:459-466.

141   **Deaths by leading cause: Deaths, by age and leading cause: 1994.**
In: *Statistical Abstract of the United States 1997*. 117th Ed. Washington, DC.
Department of Commerce. Table no. 130 p 97.

Chapter 6: Atherosclerosis

142   Kannel WB, Hjortland MC, McNamara PM, Gordon T.
Menopause and Risk of cardiovascular disease: The Framingham Study.
Ann Internal Med. 1976 Oct. 85(4):447-452.

Punnonen R, Ikalainen M, Seppala E.
Premenopausal hysterectomy and risk of cardiovascular disease.
Lancet. 1987 May 16. 1(8542):1139.

Centerwall BS.
Premenopausal hysterectomy and cardiovascular disease.
Amer Jour Obstet Gynecol. 1981 Jan 1. 139(1):58-61.

143   Wuest JH, Dry TJ, Edwards JE.
**The degree of coronary atherosclerosis in bilaterally oophorectomized
women.**
Circulation. 1953 June. 7(6):801-9.

144   Blakiston's Pocket Medical Dictionary. 3rd Ed., s.v. "atherosclerosis."

145   Blakiston's Pocket Medical Dictionary. 3rd Ed., s.v. "arteriosclerosis."

146   Kannel WB, Hjortland MC, McNamara PM, Gordon T.
Menopause and Risk of cardiovascular disease: The Framingham Study.
Ann Internal Med. 1976 Oct. 85(4):447-452.

147   Oliver MF, Edin MD, Boyd GS.
**Effect of bilateral ovariectomy on coronary-artery disease and serum-lipid
levels.**
Lancet. 1959 Oct. 2:690-4.

Clarkson TB, Anthony MS, Potvin Klein K.
Effects of estrogen treatment on arterial wall structure and function.

148   *Drugs.* 1994. 47(Suppl 2):42-51, 52-53.
148   Colditz GA, Willett WC, Stampfer JM, et al.
        Menopause and the risk of coronary heart disease in women.
        New Engl Jour Med. 1987 April. 316(18):1105-1110.

149   Silfverstolpe G, Crona N.
        Hormonal replacement therapy—cardiovascular disease.
        Acta Obstet Gynecol Scand Suppl. 1986. 134:93-95.

150   Tomita T, Sawamura F, Uetsuka R, Chiba T, Miura S, et al.
        Inhibition of cholesterylester accumulation by 17β-estradiol in macrophages
        through activation of neutral cholesterol esterase.
        Biochim Biophys Acta. 1996. 1300:210-8.

        Kannel WB, Hjortland MC, McNamara PM, Gordon T.
        Menopause and Risk of cardiovascular disease: The Framingham Study.
        Ann Internal Med. 1976 Oct. 85(4):447-452.

151   WHO Scientific Group.
        Research on the menopause. Report of a WHO scientific Group.
        Geneva. World Health Organization. Techn. Rep. Ser. 670. 1981. p44.

        Parrish HM, Carr CA, Hall DG, King TM.
        Time interval from castration in premenopausal women to development of
        excessive coronary atherosclerosis.
        Amer Jour Obstet Gynecol. 1967 Sept 15. 99(2):155-162.

152   Parrish HM, Carr CA, Hall DG, King TM.
        Time interval from castration in premenopausal women to development of
        excessive coronary atherosclerosis.
        Amer Jour Obstet Gynecol. 1967 Sept 15. 99(2):155-162.

153   Wuest JH, Dry TJ, Edwards JE.
        The degree of coronary atherosclerosis in bilaterally oophorectomized
        women.
        Circulation. 1953 June. 7(6):801-9.

154   Parrish HM, Carr CA, Hall DG, King TM.
        Time interval from castration in premenopausal women to development of
        excessive coronary atherosclerosis.
        Amer Jour Obstet Gynecol. 1967 Sept 15. 99(2):155-162.

155   Kannel WB, Hjortland MC, McNamara PM, Gordon T.
        Menopause and Risk of cardiovascular disease: The Framingham Study.
        Ann Internal Med. 1976 Oct. 85(4):447-452.

        Colditz GA, Willett WC, Stampfer JM, et al.
        Menopause and the risk of coronary heart disease in women.
        New Engl Jour Med. 1987 April. 316(18):1105-1110.

        Robinson RW, Higano N, Cohen WD.
        Increased incidence of coronary heart disease in women castrated prior to
        the menopause.
        AMA Arch Intern Med. 1959 Dec. 104:908-913.

156   Kretzschmar NR, Gardiner S.
        A consideration of the surgical menopause after hysterectomy and the
        occurrence of cancer in the stump following subtotal hysterectomy.
        Amer Jour Obstet Gynecol. 1935. 29:168-175.

        Siddle N, Sarrel P, Whitehead M.
        The effect of hysterectomy on the age at ovarian failure: identification of a
        subgroup of women with premature loss of ovarian function and literature
        review.
        Fertil Steril. 1987 Jan. 47(1):94-100.

        Dippel AL.
        The role of hysterectomy in the production of menopausal symptoms.

Amer Jour Obstet Gynecol. 1939. 37:111-3.

Sessums JV, Murphy DP.
Hysterectomy and the artificial menopause: review of literature, report of ninety-one cases.
Surg Gynecol Obstet. 1932 Jan-Mar. 54:286-9.

157   Parrish HM, Carr CA, Hall DG, King TM.
Time interval from castration in premenopausal women to development of excessive coronary atherosclerosis.
Amer Jour Obstet Gynecol. 1967 Sept 15. 99(2):155-162.

158   Pokras R, Hufnagel VG.
Hysterectomies in the United States, 1965-84: Data from the National Health Survey.
In: *Vital & Health Statistics.* Washington, DC. CDC. Series 13, number 92. pp1-31.

Whelan EA, Sandler DP, et al.
Menstrual and reproductive characteristics and age at natural menopause.
Amer Jour Epidemiol. 1990. 131(4):625-632.

National Center for Health Statistics: Utilization of short-stay hospitals: Annual summary for the United States.
In: *Vital & Health Statistics.* Washington, DC. Series 13, number 128. Table 22. p 40.

Thompson B, Hart SA, Durno D.
Menopausal age and symptomatology in general practice.
Jour Biosoc Sci. 1973. 5:71-82.

159   Wuest JH, Dry TJ, Edwards JE.
The degree of coronary atherosclerosis in bilaterally oophorectomized women.
Circulation. 1953 June. 7(6):801-9.

160   Colditz GA, Willett WC, Stampfer JM, et al.
Menopause and the risk of coronary heart disease in women.
New Engl Jour Med. 1987 April. 316(18):1105-1110.

161   Bush TL, Barrett-Connor E, Cowan LD, et al.
Cardiovascular mortality and noncontraceptive use of estrogen in women: results from the Lipid Research Clinics program follow-up study.
Circulation. 1987. 75(6):1102-9.

162   Hsueh AJW, Billig H.
Ovarian hormone synthesis and mechanism of action.
In: *Endocrinology.* ed. by DeGroot LJ, et al. 3rd ed. Philadelphia, PA. WB Saunders Co. 1995. Vol. 3. Ch. 115. p2020-1.

163   Brewer HB Jr, Santamarina-Fojo S, Hoeg JM.
Disorders of lipoprotein metabolism.
In: *Endocrinology.* ed. by DeGroot LJ, et al. 3rd ed. Philadelphia, PA. WB Saunders Co. 1995. Vol. 3. Ch. 148. p2731.

164   Glomset JA.
The plasma lecithin: cholesterol acyltransferase reaction.
Jour Lipid Res. 1968. 9:155-167.

Glomset JA, Janssen ET, et al.
Role of plasma lecithin: cholesterol acyltransferase in the metabolism of high density lipoproteins.
Jour Lipid Res. 1966. 7:638-648.

Brewer HB Jr, Santamarina-Fojo S, Hoeg JM.
Disorders of lipoprotein metabolism.
In: *Endocrinology.* ed. by DeGroot LJ, et al. 3rd ed. Philadelphia, PA. WB Saunders Co. 1995. Vol. 3. Ch. 148. pp2731-7.

165   Heiss G, Tamir I, Davis CE, et al.
        Lipoprotein-cholesterol distributions in selected North American popula-
        tions: The Lipid Research Clinics Program Prevalence Study.
        Circulation. 1980 Feb. 61(2):302-315.
        Notelovitz M, Gudat JC, Ware MD, Dougherty MC.
        Lipids and lipoproteins in women after oophorectomy and the response to
        oestrogen therapy.
        Brit Jour Obstet Gynaecol. 1983 Feb. 90:171-7.

166   Stevenson JC, Crook D, Godsland IF.
        Influence of age and menopause on serum lipids and lipoproteins in healthy
        women.
        Atherosclerosis. 1993. 98:83-90.

167   Giral P, Filitti V, Levenson J, et al.
        Relation of risk factors for cardiovascular disease to early atherosclerosis
        detected by ultrasonography in middle-aged normotensive hypercholester-
        olemic men.
        Atherosclerosis. 1990. 85:151-9.
        Punnonen R, Jokela H, Aine R, et al.
        Impaired ovarian function and risk factors for atherosclerosis in premeno-
        pausal women.
        Maturitas. 1997. 27:231-8.
        Stevenson JC, Crook D, Godsland IF.
        Influence of age and menopause on serum lipids and lipoproteins in healthy
        women.
        Atherosclerosis. 1993. 98:83-90.
        Heiss G, Tamir I, Davis CE, et al.
        Lipoprotein-cholesterol distributions in selected North American popula-
        tions: The Lipid Research Clinics Program Prevalence Study.
        Circulation. 1980 Feb. 61(2):302-315.

168   Brewer HB Jr, Santamarina-Fojo S, Hoeg JM.
        Disorders of lipoprotein metabolism.
        In: *Endocrinology.* ed. by DeGroot LJ, et al. 3rd ed. Philadelphia, PA. WB
        Saunders Co. 1995. Vol. 3. Ch. 148. p2735-6.

169   Castelo-Branco C, Casals E, et al.
        Effects of oophorectomy and hormone replacement therapy on plasma
        lipids.
        Maturitas. 1993. 17:113-122.
        Lafferty FW, Fiske ME.
        Postmenopausal estrogen replacement: a long-term cohort study.
        Amer Jour Med. 1994 Jul. 97:66-77.

170   van der Mooren MJ, Demacker PNM, et al.
        Beneficial effects on serum lipoproteins by 17β-oestradiol-dydrogesterone
        therapy in postmenopausal women; a prospective study.
        Euro Jour Obstet Gynecol Repro Biol. 1992. 47:153-160.
        Castelo-Branco C, Casals E, et al.
        Effects of oophorectomy and hormone replacement therapy on plasma
        lipids.
        Maturitas. 1993. 17:113-122.

171   Kim CJ, Jang HC, Cho DH, Min YK.
        Effects of hormone replacement therapy on lipoprotein(a) and lipids in
        postmenopausal women.

Arterioscler Thromb. 1994 Feb. 14(2):275-281.

Tonstad S, Ose L, Gorbitz C, et al.
Efficacy of sequential hormone replacement therapy in the treatment of hypercholesterolaemia among postmenopausal women.
Jour Inter Med. 1995. 238:39-47.

172   Lobo RA, Pickar JH, Wild RA, et al.
Metabolic impact of adding medroxyprogesterone acetate to conjugated estrogen therapy in postmenopausal women.
Obstet Gynecol. 1994 Dec. 84(6):987-995.

173   Lobo RA, Pickar JH, Wild RA, et al.
Metabolic impact of adding medroxyprogesterone acetate to conjugated estrogen therapy in postmenopausal women.
Obstet Gynecol. 1994 Dec. 84(6):987-995.

Silfverstolpe G, Gustafson A, Samsioe G, Svanborg A.
Lipid metabolic studies in oophorectomized women: effects induced by two different estrogens on serum lipids and lipoproteins.
Gynecol Obstet Invest. 1980. 11:161-9.

Hirvonen E, Malkonen M, Manninen V.
Effects of different progestogens on lipoproteins during postmenopausal replacement therapy.
New Engl Jour Med. 1981 Mar. 304(10):560-3.

174   Schram JHN, Boerrigter PJ, et al.
Influence of two hormone replacement therapy regimens, oral oestradiol valerate and cyproterone acetate versus transdermal oestradiol and oral dydrogesterone, on lipid metabolism.
Maturitas. 1995. 22:121-130.

175   Tikkanen MJ.
The menopause and hormone replacement therapy: lipids, lipoproteins, coagulation and fibrinolytic factors.
Maturitas. 1996. 23:209-216.

176   Castelo-Branco C, Casals E, et al.
Effects of oophorectomy and hormone replacement therapy on plasma lipids.
Maturitas. 1993. 17:113-122.

177   Clarkson TB.
Estrogens, progestins, and coronary heart disease in cynomolgus monkeys.
Fertil Steril. 1994 Dec. 62(Suppl 2)6:147S-151S.

Bush TL, Cowan LD, Barrett-Connor E, et al.
Estrogen use and all-cause mortality - Preliminary results from the Lipid Research Clinics program follow-up study.
Jour Amer Med Assoc. 1983 Feb. 249:903-6.

Stevenson JC, Crook D, Godsland IF, et al.
Hormone replacement therapy and cardiovascular system: nonlipid effects.
Drugs. 1994. 47(suppl 2):35-41.

178   Wagner JD, Clarkson TB, et al.
Estrogen and progesterone replacement therapy reduces low density lipoprotein accumulation in the coronary arteries of surgically postmenopausal cynomolgus monkeys.
Jour Clin Invest. 1991 88:1995-2002.

179   Karas RH, Patterson BL, Mendelsohn ME.
Human vascular smooth muscle cells contain functional estrogen receptor.

Circulation. 1994 May. 89(5):1943-1950.

Orimo A, Inoue S, Ikegami A, Hosoi T, et al.

Vascular smooth muscle cells as target for estrogen.

Biochem Biophys Res Comm. 1993 Sept 15. 195(2):730-6.

Knauthe R, Diel P, Hegele-Hartung C, et al.

Sexual dimorphism of steroid hormone receptor messenger ribonucleic acid expression and hormonal regulation in rat vascular tissue.

Endocrinology. 1996. 137(8):3220-7.

180   Losordo DW, Kearney M, Kim EA, et al.

Variable expression of the estrogen receptor in normal and atherosclerotic coronary arteries of premenopausal women.

Circulation. 1994 Apr. 89(4):1501-1510.

181   Muscat Baron Y, Brincat M, Galea R.

Carotid artery wall thickness in women treated with hormone replacement therapy.

Maturitas. 1997. 27:47-53.

182   Sack MN, Rader DJ, Cannon RO III.

Oestrogen and inhibition of oxidation of low-density lipoproteins in postmenopausal women.

Lancet. 1994 Jan 29. 343:269-270.

183   Wagner JD, Clarkson TB, et al.

Estrogen and progesterone replacement therapy reduces low density lipoprotein accumulation in the coronary arteries of surgically postmeno-pausal cynomolgus monkeys.

Jour Clin Invest. 1991 88:1995-2002.

184   Linman JW.

Hemorrhagic disorder.

In: *Principles of Hematology.* New York, NY. The Macmillan Co. 1966. Ch. 13. pp464-482.

Blakiston's Pocket Medical Dictionary. 3rd Ed., s.v. "fibrinogen."

185   Punnonen R, Jokela H, Aine R, et al.

Impaired ovarian function and risk factors for atherosclerosis in premeno-pausal women.

Maturitas. 1997. 27:231-8.

Heinrich J, Balleisen L, et al.

Fibrinogen and factor VII in the prediction of coronary risk: results from the PROCAM study in healthy men.

Arterioscler Thromb. 1994 Jan. 14(1):54-9.

186   Punnonen R, Jokela H, Aine R, et al.

Impaired ovarian function and risk factors for atherosclerosis in premeno-pausal women.

Maturitas. 1997. 27:231-8.

187   Espinosa E, Oemar BS, Luscher TF.

17β-estradiol and smooth muscle cell proliferation in aortic cells of male and female rats.

Biochem Biophys Res Comm. 1996. 221(1):8-14.

188   Collins P, Rosano GMC, Sarrel PM, Ulrich L, et al.

17β-Estradiol attenuates acetylcholine-induced coronary arterial constric-tion in women but not men with coronary heart disease.

Circulation. 1995 Jul 1. 92(1):24-30.

Rosano GMC, Sarrel PM, Poole-Wilson PA, Collins P.

Beneficial effect of oestrogen on exercise-induced myocardial ischaemia in women with coronary artery disease.

Lancet. 1993 Jul. 342:133-6.

Freay AD, Curtis SW, Korach KS, et al.
Mechanism of vascular smooth muscle relaxation by estrogen in depolarized rat and mouse aorta.
Circ Res. 1997 Aug. 81(2):242-8.

189   Freay AD, Curtis SW, Korach KS, et al.
Mechanism of vascular smooth muscle relaxation by estrogen in depolarized rat and mouse aorta.
Circ Res. 1997 Aug. 81(2):242-8.

190   Varma TR, Everard D, Hole D.
Effect of natural estrogen on the serum level of follicle-stimulating hormone (FSH), estradiol and estrone in post-menopausal women and its effect on endometrium.
Acta Obstet Gynecol Scand. 1985. 64:105-9.

191   Piazze Garnica JJ, Anceschi MM, et al.
Differences in erythrocyte membrane cholesterol to phospholipids ratio in postmenopausal women with and without hormone replacement.
Eur Jour Obstet Gynecol Repro Biol. 1997. 72:191-4.

192   Own JS, Bruckdorder KR, et al.
Decreased erythrocyte membrane fluidity and altered lipid composition in human liver disease.
Jour Lipid Res. 1982. 23:124-132.

Chien S.
Red cell deformability and its relevance to blood flow.
Ann Rev Physiol. 1987. 49:177-192.

Garnier M, Koutsouris D, Hanss M.
On the membrane determinant of the erythrocyte deformability.
Clin Hemorheol. 1985. 5(5):401-9.

193   Piazze Garnica JJ, Anceschi MM, et al.
Differences in erythrocyte membrane cholesterol to phospholipids ratio in postmenopausal women with and without hormone replacement.
Eur Jour Obstet Gynecol Repro Biol. 1997. 72:191-4.

194   Psaty BM, Heckbert SR, Atkins D, et al.
The risk of myocardial infarction associated with the combined use of estrogens and progestins in postmenopausal women.
Arch Intern Med. 1994 Jun 27. 154:1333-9.

195   Winkler UH.
Effects of androgens on haemostasis.
Maturitas. 1996. 24:147-155.

196   Winkler UH.
Effects of androgens on haemostasis.
Maturitas. 1996. 24:147-155.

197   Adams MR, Kaplan JR, Manuck SB, Koritnik DR, et al.
Inhibition of coronary artery atherosclerosis by 17-beta estradiol in ovariectomized monkey: Lack of an effect of added progesterone.
Arteriosclerosis. 1990 Nov/Dec. 10(6):1051-7.

198   Kushwaha RS, Lewis DS, Carey KD, McGill HC Jr.
Effects of estrogen and progesterone on plasma lipoproteins and experimental atherosclerosis in the baboon.
Arteriosclerosis Thromb. 1991 Jan-Feb. 11(1):23-31.

199   Sidney S, Petitti DB,Quesenberry CP Jr.
Myocardial infarction and the use of estrogen and estrogen-progestogen in postmenopausal women.

Ann Intern Med. 1997 Oct 1. 127(7):501-8.

200   Stampfer MJ, Colditz GA.
       Estrogen replacement therapy and coronary heart disease: a quantitative assessment of the epidemiologic evidence.
       Prev Med. 1991. 20:47-63.
       Bush TL, Barrett-Connor E, Cowan LD, et al.
       Cardiovascular mortality and noncontraceptive use of estrogen in women: results from the Lipid Research Clinics program follow-up study.
       Circulation. 1987. 75(6):1102-9.
       Barrett-Connor E.
       The menopause, hormone replacement, and cardiovascular disease: the epidemiologic evidence.
       Maturitas. 1996. 23:227-234.

201   Grady D, Rubin SM, Petitti DB, Fox CS, Black D, et al.
       Hormone therapy to prevent disease and prolong life in postmenopausal women.
       Ann Intern Med. 1992 Dec. 117(12):1016-1037.

202   Falkeborn M, Persson I, et al.
       The risk of acute myocardial infarction after oestrogen and oestrogen-progestogen replacement.
       Brit Jour Obstet Gynaecol. 1992 Oct. 99:821-8.

203   Parrish HM, Carr CA, Hall DG, King TM.
       Time interval from castration in premenopausal women to development of excessive coronary atherosclerosis.
       Amer Jour Obstet Gynecol. 1967 Sept 15. 99(2):155-162.

204   Meade TW, Berra A.
       Hormone replacement therapy and cardiovascular disease.
       Brit Med Bulletin. 1992 Apr. 48(2):276-308.

205   Centerwall BS.
       Premenopausal hysterectomy and cardiovascular disease.
       Amer Jour Obstet Gynecol. 1981 Jan 1. 139(1):58-61.

206   Shelton JD.
       Prostacyclin from the uterus and woman's cardiovascular advantage.
       Prostaglandins Leukotrienes Med. 1982. 8:459-466.

Chapter 7: Osteoporosis

207   **Fast facts on osteoporosis.**
       Washington, D.C. National Osteoporosis Foundation. 1998. (Internet).

208   Silver JJ, Einhorn TA.
       Osteoporosis and aging: current update.
       Clin Orthop Related Res. 1995 Jul. 316:10-20.

209   **Stand up to osteoporosis.**
       Washington, D.C. National Osteoporosis Foundation. Pamphlet 1995. Revised 1997.

210   Silver JJ, Einhorn TA.
       Osteoporosis and aging: current update.
       Clin Orthop Related Res. 1995 Jul. 316:10-20.

211   Manolagas SC, Jilka RL.
       Bone marrow, cytokines, and bone remodeling: emerging insights into the pathophysiology of osteoporosis.

New Engl Jour Med. 1995 Feb 2. 332(5):305-311.

Vander AJ, Sherman JH, Luciano DS.
Regulation of water and electrolyte balance.
In: *Human Physiology: The Mechanisms of Body Function.* 2nd ed. McGraw-Hill. 1975. Ch. 11. pp346-9.

212   Riggs BL, Melton LJ III.
Evidence for two distinct syndromes of involutional osteoporosis.
Amer Jour Med. 1983 Dec. 75(6):899-901.

213   Riggs BL, Melton LJ III.
Involutional osteoporosis.
New Engl Jour Med. 1986 June 26. 314(26):1676-1686.

Lindsay R, Hart DM, et al.
Prevention of spinal osteoporosis in oophorectomized women.
Lancet. 1980 Nov 29. 2:1151-4.

214   Riggs BL, Melton LJ III.
Involutional osteoporosis.
New Engl Jour Med. 1986 June 26. 314(26):1676-1686.

215   Galsworthy TD.
The mechanism of an osteoporosis center.
Orthopedic Clin North Amer. 1990 Jan. 21(1):163-9.
Updated per author fax (1998 Mar 11).

216   **Fast facts on osteoporosis.**
Washington, D.C. National Osteoporosis Foundation. 1998. (Internet).

217   Manolagas SC, Jilka RL.
Bone marrow, cytokines, and bone remodeling: emerging insights into the pathophysiology of osteoporosis.
New Engl Jour Med. 1995 Feb 2. 332(5):305-311.

Slemenda C, Longcope C, Peacock M, Hui S, Johnston CC.
Sex steroids, bone mass, and bone loss: A prospective study of pre-, peri-, and postmenopausal women.
Journ Clin Invest. 1996 Jan 1. 97(1):14-21.

218   Cann CE, Genant HK, Ettinger B, Gordan GS.
Spinal mineral loss in oophorectomized women: Determination by quantitative computed tomography.
Jour Amer Med Assoc. 1980 Nov 7. 244(18):2056-9.

219   Kreiger N, Kelsey JL, Holford TR, O'Connor T.
An epidemiologic study of hip fracture in postmenopausal women.
Amer Jour Epidemiol. 1982. 116(1):141-8.

220   Komm BS, Terpening CM, Benz DJ, et al.
Estrogen binding, receptor mRNA, and biologic response in osteoblast-like osteosarcoma cells.
Science. 1988 Jul 1. 241:81-4.

Eriksen EF, Colvard DS, et al.
Evidence of estrogen receptors in normal human osteoblast-like cells.
Science. 1988 Jul 1. 241:84-6.

Prior JC.
Progesterone as bone-trophic hormone.
Endocrine Reviews. 1990 May. 11(2):386-398.

221   Martin TJ.
Hormones in the coupling of bone resorption and formation.
Osteoporosis Int. 1993. Suppl 1:S121-5.

222   Lafferty FW, Helmuth DO.
Post-menopausal estrogen replacement: the prevention of osteoporosis and systemic effects.

Maturitas. 1985. 7:147-159.

Lindsay R, Hart DM, et al.
Prevention of spinal osteoporosis in oophorectomized women.
Lancet. 1980 Nov 29. 2:1151-4.

Lufkin EG, Wahner HW, O'Fallon WM, Hodgson SF, et al.
Treatment of postmenopausal osteoporosis with transdermal estrogen.
Ann Intern Med. 1992 July 1. 117(1):1-9.

Lindsay R, Tohme JF.
Estrogen treatment of patients with established postmenopausal osteoporo-sis.
Obstet Gynecol. 1990 Aug. 76(2):290-5.

223   Kiel DP, Felson DT, et al.
Hip fractures and the use of estrogens in postmenopausal women: The Framingham Study.
New Engl Jour Med. 1987 Nov 5. 317(19):1169-1174.

224   Lafferty FW, Helmuth DO.
Post-menopausal estrogen replacement: the prevention of osteoporosis and systemic effects.
Maturitas. 1985. 7:147-159.

225   Wei LL, Leach MW, Miner RS, Demers LM.
Evidence for progesterone receptor in human osteoblast-like cells.
Biochem Biophys Res Comm. 1993 Sept 15. 195(2):525-532.

MacNamara P, O'Shaughnessy C, Manduca P, Loughrey HC.
Pregesterone receptors are expressed in human osteoblast-like cell lines and in primary human osteoblast cultures.
Calcif Tissue Int. 1995. 57:436-441.

Prior JC.
Progesterone as bone-trophic hormone.
Endocrine Reviews. 1990 May. 11(2):386-398.

226   Lufkin EG, Wahner HW, O'Fallon WM, Hodgson SF, et al.
Treatment of postmenopausal osteoporosis with transdermal estrogen.
Ann Intern Med. 1992 July 1. 117(1):1-9.

227   Lufkin EG, Riggs BL.
Three-year follow-up on effects of transdermal estrogen.
Ann Intern Med. 1996 July 1. 125(1):77.

228   Prior JC.
Progesterone as bone-trophic hormone.
Endocrine Reviews. 1990 May. 11(2):386-398.

Lee JR.
Is natural progesterone the missing link in osteoporosis prevention and treatment?
Med Hypotheses. 1991 Aug. 35(4):316-8.

229   Wang C, Eyre DR, Clark R, Kleinberg D, Newman C, et al.
Sublingual testosterone replacement improves muscle mass and strength, decreases bone resorption, and increases bone formation markers in hypogonadal men - A Clinical Research Center Study.
Jour Clin Endocrinol Metab. 1996. 81(10):3654-3662.

Benz DJ, Haussler MR, Thomas MA, et al.
High-affinity androgen binding and androgenic regulation of a1(I)-Procollagen and transforming growth factor-b steady state messenger ribonucleic acid levels in human osteoblast-like osteosarcoma cells.

Endocrinology. 1991. 128(6):2723-2730.

230   Jassal SK, Barrett-Conner E, Edelstein SL.
       **Low bioavailable testosterone levels predict future height loss in postmeno-
       pausal women.**
       Jour Bone Mineral Res. 1995 Apr. 10(4):650-4.

231   Slemenda C, Longcope C, Peacock M, Hui S, Johnston CC.
       **Sex steroids, bone mass, and bone loss: A prospective study of pre-, peri-,
       and postmenopausal women.**
       Journ Clin Invest. 1996 Jan 1. 97(1):14-21.

232   Raisz LG.
       **Physiologic and pathologic roles of prostaglandins and other eicosanoids in
       bone metabolism.**
       Jour Nutrition. 1995. 125:2024S-2027S.

233   Vander AJ, Sherman JH, Luciano DS.
       Regulation of water and electrolyte balance.
       In: *Human Physiology: The Mechanisms of Body Function.* 2nd ed. McGraw-
       Hill. 1975. Ch. 11. pp346-9.

       Potts JT Jr, Bringhurst FR, Gardella T, et al.
       **Parathyroid hormone: physiology, chemistry, biosynthesis, secretion,
       metabolism, and mode of action.**
       In: *Endocrinology.* ed. by DeGroot LJ, et al. 3rd ed. Philadelphia, PA. WB
       Saunders Co. 1995. Vol. 2. p921.

       Tam CS, Bayley A, Cross EG, et al.
       **Increased bone apposition in primary hyperparathyroidism: measurements
       based on short interval tetracycline labeling of bone.**
       Metabolism. 1982 Aug. 31(8):759-765.

234   Vander AJ, Sherman JH, Luciano DS.
       Regulation of water and electrolyte balance.
       In: *Human Physiology: The Mechanisms of Body Function.* 2nd ed. McGraw-
       Hill. 1975. Ch. 11. p349.

235   Stevenson JC, Abeyasekera G, et al.
       **Calcitonin and the calcium-regulating hormones in postmenopausal women:
       effect of oestrogens.**
       Lancet. 1981 Mar 28. p693-5.

236   Davidson BJ, Riggs BL, Wahner HW, Judd HL.
       **Endogenous cortisol and sex steroids in patients with osteoporotic spinal
       fractures.**
       Obstet Gynecol. 1983 Mar. 61(3):275-8.

237   Breslau NA.
       Calcium, estrogen, and progestin in the treatment of osteoporosis.
       Rheum Dis Clin North Amer. 1994 Aug. 20(3):691-716.

       Orimo H, Shiraki M, Inoue S.
       Estrogen and bone.
       Osteoporosis Int. 1993. Suppl 1:S153-6.

238   Barengolts EI, Lathon PV', Lindh FG.
       **Progesterone antagonist RU 486 has bone-sparing effects in ovariectomized
       rats.**
       Bone. 1995 Jul. 17(1):21-5.

       Shen V, Birchman R, Xu R, Otter M, Wu D, Lindsay R, Dempster DW.
       **Effects of reciprocal treatment with estrogen and estrogen plus parathyroid
       hormone on bone structure and strength in ovariectomized rats.**

Journal Clin Invest. 1995 Nov. 96(5):2331-8.
Bagi C, van der Meulen M, Brommage R, Rosen D, Sommer A.
The effect of systemically administered rhIGF-I/IGFBP-3 complex on cortical bone strength and structure in ovariectomized rats.
Bone. 1995 May. 16(5):559-565.
Li M, Wronski TJ.
Response of femoral neck to estrogen depletion and parathyroid hormone in aged rats.
Bone. 1995 May. 16(5):551-7.
Kalu DN, Liu C-C, Hardin RR, Hollis BW.
The aged rat model of ovarian hormone deficiency bone loss.
Endocrinology. 1988. 124(1):7-16.
Goda T, Suruga K, Takase S, Ezawa I, Hosoya N.
Dietary maltitol increases calcium content and breaking force of femoral bone in ovariectomized rats.
Jour Nutrition. 1995. 125:2869-2873.
Yamauchi H, Kushida K, Yamazaki K, Inoue T.
Assessment of spine bone mineral density in ovariectomized rats using DXA.
Jour Bone Min Res. 1995. 10(7):1033-1039.
Beaudreuil J, Mbalaviele G, Cohen-Solal M, Morieux C, et al.
Short-term local injections of transforming growth factor-b1 decrease ovariectomy-stimulated osteoclastic resorption in vivo in rats.
Jour Bone Min Res. 1995. 10(6):971-7.
239   Yamauchi H, Kushida K, Yamazaki K, Inoue T.
Assessment of spine bone mineral density in ovariectomized rats using DXA.
Jour Bone Min Res. 1995. 10(7):1033-1039.
Wronski TJ, Dann LM, Scott KS, Cintron M.
Long-term effects of ovariectomy and aging on the rat skeleton.
Calcif Tissue Int. 1989. 45:360-6.
240   Goda T, Suruga K, Takase S, Ezawa I, Hosoya N.
Dietary maltitol increases calcium content and breaking force of femoral bone in ovariectomized rats.
Jour Nutrition. 1995. 125:2869-2873.
Kalu DN, Liu C-C, Hardin RR, Hollis BW.
The aged rat model of ovarian hormone deficiency bone loss.
Endocrinology. 1988. 124(1):7-16.
241   Krall EA, Dawson-Hughes B, Papas A, Garcia RI.
Tooth loss and skeletal bone density in healthy postmenopausal women.
Osteoporosis Int. 1994. 4:104-9.
242   Elovic RP; Hipp JA; Hyaes WC.
Maxillary molar extraction causes increased bone loss in the mandible of ovariectomized rats.
Jour Bone Min Res. 1995 Jul. 10(7):1087-1093.
243   **Fast facts on osteoporosis.**
Washington, D.C. National Osteoporosis Foundation. 1998. (Internet).
Riggs BL.
Overview of osteoporosis.
West Jour Med. 1991 Jan. 154:63-77.
244   **Fast facts on osteoporosis.**
Washington, D.C. National Osteoporosis Foundation. 1998. (Internet).
Stand up to osteoporosis.
Washington, D.C. National Osteoporosis Foundation. 1995. Rev. 1997.

(Pamphlet).

245 **Stand up to osteoporosis.**
Washington, D.C. National Osteoporosis Foundation. 1995. Rev. 1997.
(Pamphlet).

246 Beals RK.
Survival following hip fracture: long follow-up of 607 patients.
Jour Chron Dis. 1972. 25:235-244.

247 **Expectation of life: expectation of life by sex, 1985-1995.**
In: *Information Please Almanac - 1998.* ed. by Brunner B. Boston, MA.
Houghton Mifflin Co. 1997. p846.

248 Watson, NR, Studd JWW, Garnett T, Savvas M, Milligan P.
Bone loss after hysterectomy with ovarian conservation.
Obstet Gynecol. 1995 Jul. 86(1):72-7.

249 **Osteoporosis? What you should know . . . What you can do to help preserve
your independence.**
Merck Pharmaceuticals. 1995. L5670-9, 1095. (Brochure).

250 **Cutting edge reports: National osteoporosis foundation applauds inclusion of
osteoporosis test in balance budget act.**
Washington, D.C. National Osteoporosis Foundation. 1997 Aug. (Internet).

251 **Package inserts - FOSAMAX.**
West Point, PA. Merck & Co., Inc. 1997 Apr. Circular no. 7957006.

252 Silver JJ, Einhorn TA.
Osteoporosis and aging: current update.
Clin Orthop Related Res. 1995 Jul. 316:10-20.

253 Gambert SR, Schultz BM, Hamdy RC.
Osteoporosis: clinical features, prevention, and treatment.
Endocrin Metab Clin North Amer. 1995 Jun. 24(2):317-371.

254 **Stand up to osteoporosis.**
Washington, D.C. National Osteoporosis Foundation. 1995. Rev. 1997.
(Pamphlet).

Chapter 8: Weight

255 Gould D.
Hidden problems after a hysterectomy.
Nursing Times. 1986 June 4. 82(23):43-6.
Luoto R, Kaprio J, Reunanen A, Rutanen E-M.
Cardiovascular morbidity in relation to ovarian function after hysterectomy.
Obstet Gynecol. 1995 Apr. 85(4):515-522.

256 Luoto R, Kaprio J, Reunanen A, Rutanen E-M.
Cardiovascular morbidity in relation to ovarian function after hysterectomy.
Obstet Gynecol. 1995 Apr. 85(4):515-522.

257 Li M, Wronski TJ.
**Response of femoral neck to estrogen depletion and parathyroid hormone in
aged rats.**
Bone. 1995 May. 16(5):551-7.
Beaudreuil J, Mbalaviele G, Cohen-Solal M, Morieux C, et al.
**Short-term local injections of transforming growth factor-b1 decrease
ovariectomy-stimulated osteoclastic resorption in vivo in rats.**

Jour Bone Min Res. 1995. 10(6):971-7.

258   Naito Y, Fukata J, Tamai S, Seo N, Nakai Y, et al.
Biphasic changes in hypothalamo-pituitary-adrenal function during the early recovery period after major abdominal surgery.
Jour Clin Endocrinol Metab. 1991 Jul. 73(1):111-7.

259   Wilber JF.
Control of thyroid function: the hypothalamic-pituitary-thyroid axis.
In: *Endocrinology.* ed. by DeGroot LJ, et al. 3rd ed. Philadelphia, PA. WB Saunders Co. 1995. Vol. 1. Ch. 38. p609.

260   Vander AJ, Sherman JH, Luciano DS.
Regulation of organic metabolism and energy balance.
In: *Human Physiology: The Mechanisms of Body Function.* 2nd ed. McGraw-Hill. 1975. Ch. 13. pp402-5.

    Underwood LE, Van Wyk JJ.
Normal and aberrant growth.
In: *Williams Textbook of Endocrinology.* ed. by Wilson J, Foster D. 8th ed. Philadelphia, PA. WB Saunders Co. 1992. Ch. 21. p1084.

    Thorner MO, Vance ML, Horvath E, Kovacs K.
The anterior pituitary.
In: *Williams Textbook of Endocrinology.* ed. by Wilson J, Foster D. 8th ed. Philadelphia, PA. WB Saunders Co. 1992. Ch. 6. pp228-236.

261   Inzucchi SE.
Growth hormone in adults: indications and implications.
Hospital Practice. 1997 Jan 15. p79-96.

262   Jorgensen JOL, Pedersen SA, Thuesen L, et al.
Beneficial effects of growth hormone treatment in GH-deficient adults.
Lancet. 1989 June 3. 1(8649):1221-5.

263   Fazio S, Sabatini D, et al.
A preliminary study of growth hormone in the treatment of dilated cardiomyopathy.
New Engl Jour Med. 1996 Mar 28. 334(13):809-814.

264   Rosen T, Bengtsson B.
Premature mortality due to cardiovascular disease in hypopituitarism.
Lancet. 1990 Aug 4. 336:285-8.

265   De Leo V, Lanzetta D, D D'Antona, Danero S.
Growth hormone secretion in premenopausal women before and after ovariectomy: effect of hormone replacement therapy.
Fertil Steril. 1993 Aug. 60(2):268-271.

    Jansson J, Ekberg S, Isaksson OGP, Eden S.
Influence of gonadal steroids on age-and sex -related secretory patterns of growth hormone in the rat.
Endocrinology. 1984. 114(4):1287-1294.

    Frantz AG, Rabkin MT.
Effects of estrogen and sex difference on secretion of human growth hormone.
Jour Clin Endocrin. 1965 Nov. 25:1470-1480.

266   Moe KE, Prinz PN, Larsen LH, Vitiello MV, Reed SO, Merriam GR.
Growth hormone in postmenopausal women after long-term oral estrogen replacement therapy.
Jour Gerontol: Biol Sci. 1998. 53A(2):B117-B124.

267   Pringle PJ, Barton J, Fall CHD, et al.
Cortisol & growth hormone secretion in the young and the elderly.
15th Joint meeting of the British Endocrine Societies. 25-28 Mar 1996. Jour

Endocrinol. 1996 Mar. 148(Suppl):P287. (Poster).

268   Vander AJ, Sherman JH, Luciano DS.
        Defense mechanisms of the body.
        In: *Human Physiology: The Mechanisms of Body Function.* 2nd ed. McGraw-
        Hill. 1975. Ch. 15. pp499-501.

269   Bjorntorp P.
        **Growth hormone, insulin-like growth factor-I and lipid metabolism:
        interactions with sex steroids.**
        Horm Res. 1996. 46:188-191.

        Carroll PV, Christ ER, et al.
        **Growth hormone deficiency in adulthood and the effects of growth hormone
        replacement: a review.**
        Jour Clin Endocrinol Metab. 1998. 83(2):382-395.

        Vander AJ, Sherman JH, Luciano DS.
        Regulation of organic metabolism and energy balance.
        In: *Human Physiology: The Mechanisms of Body Function.* 2nd ed. McGraw-
        Hill. 1975. Ch. 13. pp402-421.

        Underwood LE, Van Wyk JJ.
        Normal and aberrant growth.
        In: *Williams Textbook of Endocrinology.* ed. by Wilson J, Foster D. 8th ed.
        Philadelphia, PA. WB Saunders Co. 1992. Ch. 21. p1084.

        Thorner MO, Vance ML, Horvath E, Kovacs K.
        The anterior pituitary.
        In: *Williams Textbook of Endocrinology.* ed. by Wilson J, Foster D. 8th ed.
        Philadelphia, PA. WB Saunders Co. 1992. Ch. 6. pp228-236.

270   DeFronzo RA, Ferrannini E.
        Regulation of intermediary metabolism during fasting and feeding.
        In: *Endocrinology.* ed. by DeGroot LJ, et al. 3rd ed. Philadelphia, PA. WB
        Saunders Co. 1995. Vol. 2. Ch 81. p1406.

        Flier JS.
        Syndromes of insulin resistance and mutant insulin.
        In: *Endocrinology.* ed. by DeGroot LJ, et al. 3rd ed. Philadelphia, PA. WB
        Saunders Co. 1995. Vol. 2. Ch. 91. p1593.

271   Poretsky L.
        **On the paradox of insulin-induced hyperandrogenism in insulin-resistant
        states.**
        Endocr Rev. 1991. 12(1):3-13.

272   Vander AJ, Sherman JH, Luciano DS.
        Energy and cellular metabolism.
        In: *Human Physiology: The Mechanisms of Body Function.* 2nd ed. McGraw-
        Hill. 1975. Ch. 3. pp77-89.

273   Moller DE, Flier JS.
        Insulin resistance - mechanisms, syndromes, and implications.
        New Engl Jour Med. 1991 Sep 26. 325(13):938-948.

274   Olefsky JM.
        Diabetes mellitus (type II): etiology and pathogenesis.
        In: *Endocrinology.* ed. by DeGroot LJ, et al. 3rd ed. Philadelphia, PA. WB
        Saunders Co. 1995. Vol. 2. Ch. 84. pp1436-1463.

275   Reaven GM.
        Role of insulin resistance in human disease.
        Diabetes. 1988 Dec. 37:1595-1607.

        Winocour PH, Kaluvya S, Ramaiya K, et al.
        **Relation between insulinemia, body mass index, and lipoprotein composition
        in healthy, nondiabetic men and women.**

ArteriosclerThromb. 1992 Mar. 12(3):393-402.

Peiris AN, Sothmann MS, et al.

Adiposity, fat distribution, and cardiovascular risk.

Annals Internal Med. 1989 Jun 1. 110(11):867-872.

Shinozaki K, Hattori Y, Suzuki M, et al.

Insulin resistance as an independent risk factor for carotid artery wall intima media thickening in vasospastic angina.

Arterioscl Thromb Vasc Biol. 1997 Nov. 17(11):3302-3310.

276   Walton C, Godsland IF, et al.

The effects of the menopause on insulin sensitivity, secretion and elimination in non-obese, healthy women.

Eur Jour Clin Invest. 1993. 23:466-473.

Winocour PH, Kaluvya S, Ramaiya K, et al.

Relation between insulinemia, body mass index, and lipoprotein composition in healthy, nondiabetic men and women.

ArteriosclerThromb. 1992 Mar. 12(3):393-402.

277   Senoz S, Direm B, Gulekli B, Gokmen O.

Estrogen deprivation, rather than age, is responsible for the poor lipid profile and carbohydrate metabolism in women.

Maturitas. 1996. 25:107-114.

278   Kumagai S, Holmang A, Bjorntorp P.

The effects of oestrogen and progesterone on insulin sensitivity in female rats.

Acta Physiol Scand. 1993. 149:91-7.

279   Silfverstolpe G, Gustafson A, Samsioe G, Svanborg A.

Lipid metabolic studies in oophorectomized women: effects induced by two different estrogens on serum lipids and lipoproteins.

Gynecol Obstet Invest. 1980. 11:161-9.

280   Kumagai S, Holmang A, Bjorntorp P.

The effects of oestrogen and progesterone on insulin sensitivity in female rats.

Acta Physiol Scand. 1993. 149:91-7.

281   Kritz-Silverstein D, Barrett-Connor E, Wingard DL.

Hysterectomy, oophorectomy, and heart disease risk factors in older women.

Amer Jour Public Health. 1997 April. 87(4):676-680.

282   Pedersen SB, Borglum JD, et al.

Relationship between sex hormones, body composition and metabolic risk parameters in premenopausal women.

Eur Jour Endocrin. 1995. 133:200-6.

283   Pedersen SB, Borglum JD, et al.

Relationship between sex hormones, body composition and metabolic risk parameters in premenopausal women.

Eur Jour Endocrin. 1995. 133:200-6.

284   Peiris AN, Sothmann MS, et al.

Adiposity, fat distribution, and cardiovascular risk.

Annals Internal Med. 1989 Jun 1. 110(11):867-872.

Carey DG, Jenkins AB, et al.

Abdominal fat and insulin resistance in normal and overweight women: direct measurements reveal a strong relationship in subjects at both low and high risk of NIDDM.

Diabetes. 1996 May. 45:633-8.

285   Van Cauter E, Turek FW.

Endocrine and other biological rhythms.

In: *Endocrinology.* ed. by DeGroot LJ, et al. 3rd ed. Philadelphia, PA. WB

Saunders Co. 1995. Vol 3. Ch. 140. pp2487-2548.

286   Van Cauter E, Turek FW.
        Endocrine and other biological rhythms.
        In: *Endocrinology.* ed. by DeGroot LJ, et al. 3rd ed. Philadelphia, PA. WB
        Saunders Co. 1995. Vol 3. Ch. 140. p2502.

287   Ho KY, Evans WS, Blizzard, RM, et al.
        Effects of sex and age on the 24-hour profile of growth hormone secretion in
        man: importance of endogenous estradiol concentrations.
        Jour Clin Endocrinol Metab. 1987. 64(1):51-8.

288   Van Cauter E, Turek FW.
        Endocrine and other biological rhythms.
        In: *Endocrinology.* ed. by DeGroot LJ, et al. 3rd ed. Philadelphia, PA. WB
        Saunders Co. 1995. Vol 3. Ch. 140. pp2487-2548.

        Ho KY, Evans WS, Blizzard, RM, et al.
        Effects of sex and age on the 24-hour profile of growth hormone secretion in
        man: importance of endogenous estradiol concentrations.
        Jour Clin Endocrinol Metab. 1987. 64(1):51-8.

289   Goldman JA, Reichman J, Resnik R.
        Age-related glucose metabolism alterations in nondiabetic and potentially
        diabetic women.
        Maturitas. 1980. 2:119-124.

290   Rincon J, Holmang A, et al.
        Mechanisms behind insulin resistance in rat skeletal muscle after oophorec-
        tomy and additional testosterone treatment.
        Diabetes. 1996 May. 45:615-621.

291   Ho KY, Evans WS, Blizzard, RM, et al.
        Effects of sex and age on the 24-hour profile of growth hormone secretion in
        man: importance of endogenous estradiol concentrations.
        Jour Clin Endocrinol Metab. 1987. 64(1):51-8.

        Moe KE, Prinz PN, Larsen LH, Vitiello MV, Reed SO, Merriam GR.
        Growth hormone in postmenopausal women after long-term oral estrogen
        replacement therapy.
        Jour Gerontol: Biol Sci. 1998. 53A(2):B117-B124.

        Mercuri N, Petraglia F, Genazzani AD, et al.
        Hormonal treatments modulate pulsatile plasma growth hormone, gonadot-
        rophin and osteocalcin levels in postmenopausal women.
        Maturitas. 1993. 17:51-62.

        Friend KE, Hartman ML, et al.
        Both oral and transdermal estrogen increase growth hormone release in
        postmenopausal women - a clinical research center study.
        Jour Clin Endocrinol Metab. 1996. 81(6):2250-6.

        Rodriguez-Arnao J, Perry L, et al.
        Growth hormone treatment in hypopituitary GH deficient adults reduces
        circulating cortisol levels during hydrocortisone replacement therapy.
        Clin Endocrinol. 1996. 45:33-7.

        Vander AJ, Sherman JH, Luciano DS.
        Defense mechanisms of the body.
        In: *Human Physiology: The Mechanisms of Body Function.* 2nd ed. McGraw-
        Hill. 1975. Ch. 15. pp499-502.

        Johnston DG, Gill A, et al.
        Metabolic effects of cortisol in man - studies with somatostatin.

Metabolism. 1982 April. 31(4):312-7.

Walton C, Godsland IF, et al.

The effects of the menopause on insulin sensitivity, secretion and elimination in non-obese, healthy women.

Eur Jour Clin Invest. 1993. 23:466-473.

Rincon J, Holmang A, et al.

Mechanisms behind insulin resistance in rat skeletal muscle after oophorectomy and additional testosterone treatment.

Diabetes. 1996 May. 45:615-621.

Kritz-Silverstein D, Barrett-Connor E, Wingard DL.

Hysterectomy, oophorectomy, and heart disease risk factors in older women.

Amer Jour Public Health. 1997 April. 87(4):676-680.

Samra JS, Clark ML, et al.

Effects of physiological hypercortisolemia on the regulation of lipolysis in subcutaneous adipose tissue.

Jour Clin Endocrinol Metab. 1998. 83(2):626-631.

Winocour PH, Kaluvya S, Ramaiya K, et al.

Relation between insulinemia, body mass index, and lipoprotein composition in healthy, nondiabetic men and women.

ArteriosclerThromb. 1992 Mar. 12(3):393-402.

Senoz S, Direm B, Gulekli B, Gokmen O.

Estrogen deprivation, rather than age, is responsible for the poor lipid profile and carbohydrate metabolism in women.

Maturitas. 1996. 25:107-114.

Underwood LE, Van Wyk JJ.

Normal and aberrant growth.

In: *Williams Textbook of Endocrinology.* ed. by Wilson J, Foster D. 8th ed. Philadelphia, PA. WB Saunders Co. 1992. Ch. 21. p1084.

Thorner MO, Vance ML, Horvath E, Kovacs K.

The anterior pituitary.

In: *Williams Textbook of Endocrinology.* ed. by Wilson J, Foster D. 8th ed. Philadelphia, PA. WB Saunders Co. 1992. Ch. 6. pp228-236.

Chapter 9: Depression

292   Richards DH.

Depression after hysterectomy.

Lancet. 1973 Aug 25. 2(7826):430-3.

Oldenhave A, Jaszmann LJB, Everaerd W, Haspels AA.

Hysterectomized women with ovarian conservation report more severe climacteric complaints than do normal climacteric women of similar age.

Amer Jour Obstet Gynecol. 1993 Mar. 168(3 pt 1):765-771.

Melody GF.

Depressive reactions following hysterectomy.

Amer Jour Obstet Gynecol. 1962 Feb 1. 83(3):410-3.

Barker MG.

Psychiatric illness after hysterectomy.

Brit Med Jour. 1968 April 13. 2:91-5.

Roopnarinesingh S, Gopeesingh T.

Hysterectomy and its psychological aftermath.

West Ind Med Jour. 1982. 31:131-4.

Richards DH.
A post-hysterectomy syndrome.
Lancet. 1974 Oct 26. 983-5.

Kaufert PA, Gilbert P, Tate R.
The Manitoba project: a re-examination of the link between menopause and depression.
Maturitas. 1992. 14:143-155.

293   Chakravarti S, Collins WP, Newton JR, Oram DH, Studd JWW.
Endocrine changes and symptomatology after oophorectomy in premenopausal women.
Brit Jour Obstet Gynaecol. 1977 Oct. 84:769-775.

294   Richards DH.
A post-hysterectomy syndrome.
Lancet. 1974 Oct 26. 983-5.

Gould D.
Hidden problems after a hysterectomy.
Nursing Times. 1986 June 4. 82(23):43-6.

295   Gould D.
Recovery from hysterectomy.
Practitioner. 1986 Sept. 230:756-7.

Drummond J, Field P.
Emotional and sexual sequelae following hysterectomy.
Health Care Women Int. 1984. 5: 261-271.

Turpin TJ, Heath DS.
The link between hysterectomy and depression.
Can Jour Psychiatry. 1979 Apr. 24(3): 247-254.

296   Newton N, Baron E.
Reactions to hysterectomy: Fact or fiction?
Primary Care. 1976 Dec. 3(4):781-801.

297   Howkins J, Williams D.
Total abdominal hysterectomy: 1,000 consecutive, unselected operations.
Jour Obstet Gyn Brit Common. 1963. 70:20-8.

298   Turpin TJ, Heath DS.
The link between hysterectomy and depression.
Can Jour Psychiatry. 1979 Apr. 24(3): 247-254.

299   Borell U. Fernstrom I.
The adnexal branches of the uterine artery - An arteriographic study in human subjects.
Acta Radiol. 1953 Jul. 40:561-582.

300   Siddle N, Sarrel P, Whitehead M.
The effect of hysterectomy on the age at ovarian failure: identification of a subgroup of women with premature loss of ovarian function and literature review.
Fertil Steril. 1987 Jan. 47(1):94-100.

301   Gath D, Cooper P, Bond A, Edmonds G.
Hysterectomy and psychiatric disorder: II. Demographic psychiatric and physical factors in relation to psychiatric outcome.
Brit Jour Psychiat. 1982. 140:343-350.

302   Michelson D, Stratakis C, et al.
Bone mineral density in women with depression.

New Engl Jour Med. 1996 Oct 17. 335(16):1176-1181.

303 Paschall N, Newton N.
Personality factors and postpartum adjustment.
Primary Care. 1976 Dec. 3(4):741-750.

304 Harris B, Lovett L, et al.
Maternity blues and major endocrine changes: Cardiff puerperal mood and hormone study II.
BMJ. 1994 April 9. 308:949-953.

Harris B.
Biological and hormonal aspects of postpartum depressed mood: working towards strategies for prophylaxis and treatment.
Brit Jour Psychiatry. 1994. 164:288-292.

305 Wieck A.
Endocrine aspects of postnatal mental disorders.
Bailliere's Clin Obstet Gynaecol. 1989 Dec. 3(4):857-877.

306 Pansini F, Albertazzi P, Bonaccorsi G, et al.
The menopausal transition: a dynamic approach to the pathogenesis of neurovegetative complaints.
Eur Jour Obstet Gynecol Reprod Biol. 1994 Nov. 57(2):103-9.

307 Shaver JLF.
Beyond hormonal therapies in menopause.
Exper Gerontol. 1994. 29(3/4):469-476.

Attali G, Weizman A, Gil-Ad I, Rehavi M.
Opposite modulatory effects of ovarian hormones on rat brain dopamine and serotonin transporters.
Brain Res. 1997. 756:153-9.

Coppen A, Wood K.
Tryptophan and depressive illness.
Psychological Med. 1978. 8:49-57.

Thomson J.
Double blind study on the effect of oestrogen on sleep, anxiety and depression in perimenopausal women: preliminary results.
Proc. Roy Soc Med. 1976 Nov. 69:829-830.

Casper RF, Alapin-Rubillovitz S.
Progestins increase endogenous opioid peptide activity in postmenopausal women.
Jour Clin Endocrinol Metab. 1985. 60(1):34-6.

308 Sapolsky RM.
Neuroendocrinology of the stress-response.
In: *Behavioral Endocrinology.* ed. by Becker JB, et al. Cambridge, MA. MIT Press. 1992. Chapter 10. p301-2.

309 Imura H.
Adrenocorticotrophic hormone.
In: *Endocrinology.* ed. by DeGroot LJ, et al. 3rd ed. Philadelphia, PA. WB Saunders Co. 1995. Vol. 1. Ch. 22. p362.

Reichlin S.
Neuroendocrinology.
In: *Williams Textbook of Endocrinology.* ed. by Wilson J, Foster D. 8th ed. Philadelphia, PA. WB Saunders Co. 1992. Ch. 5. pp196-9.

310 Genazzani AR, Trentini GP, Petraglia F, De Gaetani CF, et al.
Estrogens modulate the circadian rhythm of hypothalamic beta-endorphin contents in female rats.

Neuroendocrinology. 1990 Sept. 52(3):221-4.

311   Genazzani AR, Facchinetti F, Ricci-Danero MG, Parrini D, et al.
Beta-lipotropin and beta-endorphin in physiological and surgical meno-pause.
Jour Endocrinol Invest. 1981 Oct. 4(4):375-8.

312   Wardlaw SL, Wehrenberg WB, Ferin M, et al.
Effect of sex steroids on b-endorphins in hypophyseal portal blood.
Jour Clin Endocrinol Metab. 1982. 55(5):877-881.

313   Casper RF, Alapin-Rubillovitz S.
Progestins increase endogenous opioid peptide activity in postmenopausal women.
Jour Clin Endocrinol Metab. 1985. 60(1):34-6.

314   Genazzani AR, Trentini GP, Petraglia F, De Gaetani CF, et al.
Estrogens modulate the circadian rhythm of hypothalamic beta-endorphin contents in female rats.
Neuroendocrinology. 1990 Sept. 52(3):221-4.

315   Black's Medical Dictionary. 38th Ed., s.v. "serotonin."

316   Bray GA.
The syndromes of obesity: an endocrine approach.
In: *Endocrinology*. ed. by DeGroot LJ, et al. 3rd ed. Philadelphia, PA. WB Saunders Co. 1995. Vol. 3. Ch. 143. p2653.

Boucek RJ.
Serotonin and collagen metabolism.
In: *Serotonin in Health and Disease Volume IV: Clinical Correlates*. ed by Essman WB. New York. Spectrum Publications, Inc. 1977. Vol. 4. p31.

Vandermaerlen CP.
Serotonin.
In: *Neurotransmitter actions in the vertebrate nervous system*. ed. by Rogawski MA, Barker JL. New York. Plenum Press. 1985. Chapter 7. pp201-240.

317   Tuck JR, Punell G.
Uptake of [3H]5-hydroxytrptamine and [3H]noradrenaline by slices of rat brain incubated in plasma from patients treated with chlorimipramine, imipramine or amitriptyline.
Jour Pharm Pharmac. 1973. 25:573-4.

Parnate®
In: *Physicians' Desk Reference*. 52nd edition. Montvale, NJ. Medical Economics Company, Inc. 1998. p2849.

318   Fernstrom JD.
Brain serotonin and nutrition.
In: *Serotonin in health and disease. Vol. 3: The central nervous system*. ed. by Essman WB. New York. Spectrum Publications, Inc. 1978. Vol 3. p2.

319   Thomson J, Maddock J, Aylward M, Oswald I.
Relationship between nocturnal plasma oestrogen concentration and free plasma tryptophan in perimenopausal women.
Jour Endocrin. 1977. 72:395-96.

McMenamy RH, Oncley JL.
The specific binding of L-tryptophan to serum albumin.
Jour Biol Chem. 1958 Dec. 233(6):1436-1447.

320   Burton RM, Westphal U.
Steroid hormone-binding proteins in blood plasma.
Metabolism. 1972 Mar. 21(3):253-276.

321   Thomson J, Maddock J, Aylward M, Oswald I.
Relationship between nocturnal plasma oestrogen concentration and free plasma tryptophan in perimenopausal women.

Jour Endocrin. 1977. 72:395-96.

Aylward M, Maddock J.
Total and free-plasma tryptophan concentrations in rheumatoid disease.
Jour Pharm Pharmac. 1973. 25:570-2.

322   Aylward M, Maddock J.
Total and free-plasma tryptophan concentrations in rheumatoid disease.
Jour Pharm Pharmac. 1973. 25:570-2.

323   Reichlin S.
Endocrine-immune interaction.
In: *Endocrinology.* ed. by DeGroot LJ, et al. 3rd ed. Philadelphia, PA. WB
Saunders Co. 1995. Vol. 3. Ch. 158. p2977-8.

324   Vander AJ, Sherman JH, Luciano DS.
Reproduction.
In: *Human Physiology: The Mechanisms of Body Function.* 2nd ed. McGraw-
Hill. 1975. Ch. 14. pp455.

325   Reichlin S.
Endocrine-immune interaction.
In: *Endocrinology.* ed. by DeGroot LJ, et al. 3rd ed. Philadelphia, PA. WB
Saunders Co. 1995. Vol. 3. Ch. 158. pp2977-8.

326   Luine VN, Khylchevskaya RI, McEwen BS.
**Effect of gonadal steroids on activities of monoamine oxidase and choline
acetylase in rat brain.**
Brain Res. 1975. 86:293-306.

Klaiber EL, Kobayashi Y, Broverman DM, Hall F.
**Plasma monoamine oxidase activity in regularly menstruating women and in
amenorrheic women receiving cyclic treatment with estrogens and a
progestin.**
Jour Clin Endorcr. 1971. 33:630-8.

327   Sherwin BB, Gelfand MM.
**Sex steroids and affect in the surgical menopause: a double-blind, cross-over
study.**
Psychoneuroendocrinology. 1985. 10(3):325-335.

Ortega-Corona BG, Valencia-Sanchez A, et al.
**Hypothalamic monoamine oxidase activity in ovariectomized rats after
sexual behavior restoration.**
Arch Med Res. 1994. 25(3):337-340.

328   **Nardil®**
In: *Physicians' Desk Reference.* 52nd edition. Montvale, NJ. Medical Economics
Company, Inc. 1998. p2108.

Parnate®
In: *Physicians' Desk Reference.* 52nd edition. Montvale, NJ. Medical Economics
Company, Inc. 1998. p2849.

329   Fink G, Sumner BEH, Rosie R, Grace O, et al.
**Estrogen control of central neurotransmission: effect on mood, mental state,
and memory.**
Cell Molecul Neurobiol. 1996. 16(3):325-44.

330   Traskman L, Asberg M, Bertilsson L, Sjostrand L.
Monamine metabolites in CSF and suicidal behavior.
Arch Gen Psychiatry. 1981 June. 38:631-6.

Halbreich U.
Gonadal hormones and antihormones, serotonin and mood.
Psychopharmacology Bulletin. 1990. 26(3):291-6.

Weyler W, Hsu YP, Breakefield XO.
Biochemistry and genetics of monoamine oxidase.
In: *International Encyclopedia of Pharmacology and Therapeutics: Pharmaco-genetics of drug metabolism.* ed. by Kalow W. 1st ed. New York, Pergamon Press. 1992. p346-356.

Breakefield XO, Edelstein SB, Grossman MH.
Variations in MAO and NGF in cultured human skin fibroblasts.
In: *Genetic Research Strategies For Psychobiology and Psychiatry.* ed. by Gershon ES, et al. Pacific Grove, CA. Boxwood Press. 1981. Vol 1. Ch 10. pp129-142.

Murphy DL, Wright C, Buchsbaum M, et al.
Platelet and plasma amine oxidase activity in 680 normals: sex and age differences and stability over time.
Biochem Med. 1976. 16:254-265.

331 Traskman L, Asberg M, Bertilsson L, Sjostrand L.
Monamine metabolites in CSF and suicidal behavior.
Arch Gen Psychiatry. 1981 June. 38:631-6.

332 Guicheney P, Leger D, Barrat J, Trevoux R, De Lignieres B, et al.
Platelet serotonin content and plasma tryptophan in peri- and postmeno-pausal women: variations with plasma oestrogen levels and depressive symptoms.
Eur Jour Clin Invest. 1988. 18:297-304.

333 Sherwin BB, Gelfand MM.
Sex steroids and affect in the surgical menopause: a double-blind, cross-over study.
Psychoneuroendocrinology. 1985. 10(3):325-335.

334 Ditkoff EC, Crary WG, Cristo M, Lobo RA.
Estrogen improves psychological function in asymptomatic postmenopausal women.
Obstet Gynecol. 1991 Dec. 78(6):991-5.

335 Barker MG.
Psychiatric illness after hysterectomy.
Brit Med Jour. 1968 April 13. 2:91-5.

336 A Dictionary of Psychological Medicine. 1892. Vol II. s.v. "Ovariotomy and oophorectomy in relation to insanity an epilepsy."
Bantock GG
Hysterectomy and insanity.
Brit Med Jour. 1889 Aug 17. 2:395-6.

337 Ananth J.
Hysterectomy and depression.
Obstet Gynecol. 1978 Dec. 52(6):724-730.

338 **New approaches to PMS.**
In: *Harvard Women's Health Watch.* Boston, MA. Harvard Health Publications Group. 1998 Feb. V(6):6.

Chapter 10:   Fibromyalgia Syndrome

339 Goldenberg DL.
Fibromyalgia, chronic fatigue syndrome, and myofascial pain.
Cur Opin Rheumatol. 1996. 8:113-123.
The facts about chronic fatigue syndrome.
Atlanta, GA. Centers for Disease Control and Prevention. Updated Oct. 7, 1996.

(Internet).

340   Bennett R.
        **Fibromyalgia Syndrome: An informational guide for FMS patients, their
        families, friends and employers.**
        Salem, OR. National Fibromyalgia Research Assoc. June 1998. (Internet).

341   Ferraccioli G, Cavalieri F, et al.
        **Neuroendocrinologic findings in primary fibromyalgia (soft tissue chronic
        pain syndrome) and in other chronic rheumatic conditions (rheumatoid
        arthritis, low back pain).**
        Jour Rheumatol. 1990. 17(7):869-873.
        Crofford LJ, Pillemer SR, et al.
        **Hypothalamic-pituitary-adrenal axis perturbations in patients with
        fibromyalgia.**
        Arthritis Rheumatism. 1994 Nov. 37(11):1583-1592.
        Griep EN, Boersma JW, de Kloet ER.
        **Altered reactivity of the hypothalamic-pituitary-adrenal axis in the primary
        fibromyalgia syndrome.**
        Jour Rheumatol. 1993. 20:469-474.

342   Forsling ML, Anderson CHM, Wheeler MJ, Raju KS.
        **The effect of oophorectomy and hormone replacement on neurohypophyseal
        hormone secretion in women.**
        Clin Endocrinol. 1996. 44:39-44.

343   Crofford LJ, Demitrack MA.
        **Evidence that abnormalities of central neurohormonal systems are key to
        understanding fibromyalgia and chronic fatigue syndrome.**
        Rheumatic Disease Clin North Amer. 1996 May. 22(2):267-284.
        Fedor-Freybergh P.
        **The influence of oestrogens on the wellbeing and mental performance in
        climacteric and postmenopausal women.**
        Acta Obstet Gyn Scand. 1977. 64(S):1-68.

344   Bennett RM, Clark SC, Walczyk J.
        **A randomized, double-blind, placebo-controlled study of growth hormone in
        the treatment of fibromyalgia.**
        Amer Jour Med. 1998 Mar. 104:227-231.

345   Crofford LJ, Pillemer SR, et al.
        **Hypothalamic-pituitary-adrenal axis perturbations in patients with
        fibromyalgia.**
        Arthritis Rheumatism. 1994 Nov. 37(11):1583-1592.
        McCain GA, Tilbe KS.
        **Diurnal hormone variation in fibromyalgia syndrome: a comparison with
        rheumatoid arthritis.**
        Jour Rheumatol. 1989. (Suppl 19)16:154-7.

346   Russell IJ, Michalek JE, et al.
        **Platelet 3H-imipramine uptake receptor density and serum serotonin levels
        in patients with fibromyalgia/fibrositis syndrome.**
        Jour Rheumatol. 1992. 19(1):104-9.

347   Moldofsky H, Warsh JJ.
        **Plasma tryptophan and musculoskeletal pain in non-articular rheumatism
        ("Fibrositis Syndrome").**
        Pain. 1978. 5:65-71.

348   Voderholzer U, Hornyak M, et al.
        **Impact of experimentally induced serotonin deficiency by tryptophan
        depletion on sleep EEG in healthy subjects.**

Neuropsychopharmacology. 1998. 18(2):112-124.

349   Caruso I, Sarzi Puttini P, Cazzola M, Azzolini V.
Double-blind study of 5-Hydroxytryptophan versus placebo in the treatment of primary fibromyalgia syndrome.
Jour Inter Med Res. 1990. 18:201-9.

350   Niclolodi M, Sicuteri F.
Fibromyalgia and migraine, two faces of the same mechanism: serotonin as the common clue for pathogenesis and therapy.
In: *Recent advances in tryptophan research: tryptophan and serotonin pathways.* ed by Filippini GA, et al. New York. Plenum Press. 1996. Vol 398 pp373-9.

351   Crofford LJ, Demitrack MA.
Evidence that abnormalities of central neurohormonal systems are key to understanding fibromyalgia and chronic fatigue syndrome.
Rheumatic Disease Clin North Amer. 1996 May. 22(2):267-284.

352   Hakverdi AU, Taner CE, Erden AC, Satici O.
Changes in ovarian function after tubal sterilization.
Adv Contracept. 1994 Mar. 10(1):51-6.
DeStefano F, Perlman JA, Peterson HB, et al.
Long-term risk of menstrual disturbances after tubal sterilization.
Amer Jour Obstet Gynecol. 1985 Aug 1. 152(7Pt1):835-841.
Radwanska E, Headley SK, Dmowski P.
Evaluation of ovarian function after tubal sterilization.
Jour Reprod Med. 1982 July. 27(7):376-384.

353   **National Center for Health Statistics: Utilization of short-stay hospitals: Annual summary for the United States.**In: *Vital & Health Statistics.* Washington, DC. Series 13, number 128. Table 22. p 40.

Chapter 11:   Bladder and Bowel Problems

354   Smith PH, Ballantyne B.
The neuroanatomical basis for denervation of the urinary bladder following major pelvic surgery.
Brit Jour Surg. 1968 Dec. 55(12):929-933.

355   Kilkku P.
Supravaginal uterine amputation versus hysterectomy with reference to subjective bladder symptoms and incontinence.
Acta Obstet Gynecol Scand. 1985. 64:375-9.

356   Parys BT, Haylen BT, Hutton JL, Parsons KF.
The effects of simple hysterectomy on vesicourethral function.
Brit Jour Urol. 1989. 64:594-9.

357   Brown JS, Seeley DG, et al.
Urinary incontinence in older women: who is at risk?
Obstet Gynecol. 1996 May. 87(5)(part 1):715-721.

358   Parys BT, Haylen BT, Hutton JL, Parsons KF.
The effects of simple hysterectomy on vesicourethral function.
Brit Jour Urol. 1989. 64:594-9.

359   Rowe JW, Besdine RW, et al.
Urinary incontinence in adults.
National Institutes of Health Consensus Development Conference Statement. Bethesda, MD. Nat'l Inst Health. US Gov't Printing Office. 1988 Oct 3-5. Vol.

7(5):1-11.

360 De Juana CP, Everett JC Jr.
Interstitial cystitis: experience and review of recent literature.
Urology. 1977 Oct. X(4):325-9.
Koziol JA, Clark DC, Gittes RF, Tan EM.
The natural history of interstitial cystitis: a survey of 374 patients.
Jour Urology. 1993 Mar. 149:465-9.

361 Koziol JA, Clark DC, Gittes RF, Tan EM.
The natural history of interstitial cystitis: a survey of 374 patients.
Jour Urology. 1993 Mar. 149:465-9.

362 Koziol JA, Clark DC, Gittes RF, Tan EM.
The natural history of interstitial cystitis: a survey of 374 patients.
Jour Urology. 1993 Mar. 149:465-9.

363 De Juana CP, Everett JC Jr.
Interstitial cystitis: experience and review of recent literature.
Urology. 1977 Oct. X(4):325-9.

364 Alagiri M, Chottiner S, et al.
Interstitial cystitis: unexplained associations with other chronic disease and pain syndromes.
Urology. 1997. 49(suppl 5A):52-7.

365 Hanno P.
Interstitial cystitis and related diseases.
In: *Campbell's Urology.* ed. by Walsh PC, Retik AB, et al. 7th ed. Philadelphia, PA. W.B. Saunders Company. 1998. Vol 1. p642.

366 van Dam JH, Gosselink MJ, et al.
Changes in bowel function after hysterectomy.
Dis Colon Rectum. 1997. 40:1342-7.

367 Wiersma TjG, Werre AJ, et al.
Hysterectomy: the anorectal pitfall.
Scand Jour Gastroenterol. 1997. 32(suppl)223:3-7.

368 Heaton KW, Parker D, Cripps H.
Bowel function and irritable bowel symptoms after hysterectomy and cholecystectomy - a population based study.
Gut. 1993. 34:1108-1111.
Taylor T, Smith AN, et al.
Effect of hysterectomy on bowel function.
BMJ. 1989. 299:300-1.
Prior A, Stanley KM, Smith ARB, Read NW.
Relation between hysterectomy and the irritable bowel: a prospective study.
Gut. 1992 Jun. 33(6):814-7.
Smith AN, Varma JS, et al.
Disordered colorectal motility in intractable constipation following hysterectomy.
Brit Jour Surg. 1990 Dec. 77:1361-6.

369 van Dam JH, Gosselink MJ, et al.
Changes in bowel function after hysterectomy.
Dis Colon Rectum. 1997. 40:1342-7.

370 van Dam JH, Gosselink MJ, et al.
Changes in bowel function after hysterectomy.
Dis Colon Rectum. 1997. 40:1342-7.

371 Smith AN, Varma JS, et al.
Disordered colorectal motility in intractable constipation following hysterectomy.

Brit Jour Surg. 1990 Dec. 77:1361-6.

372 Taylor T, Smith AN, et al.
Effect of hysterectomy on bowel function.
BMJ. 1989. 299:300-1.

373 Smith AN, Varma JS, et al.
Disordered colorectal motility in intractable constipation following hysterectomy.
Brit Jour Surg. 1990 Dec. 77:1361-6.

374 Preston DM, Rees LH, Lennard-Jones JE.
Gynaecological disorders and hyperporlactinaemia in chronic constipation.
Gut. 1983. 24:A480:F17. (Poster).

Singh S, Poulsom R. et al.
Cyclical constipation, is it mediated by sex steroids? Gastroenterology. 1992 April. 102(4 Part 2):A515. (Poster).

375 Whitehead WE, Cheskin LJ, et al.
Evidence for exacerbation of irritable bowel syndrome during menses.
Gastroenterology. 1990 Jun. 98(6):1485-1489.

Heitkemper MM, Shaver JF, Mitchell ES.
Gastrointestinal symptoms and bowel patterns across the menstrual cycle in dysmenorrhea.
Nursing Res. 1988 Mar-Apr. 37(2):108-113.

376 Whitehead WE, Cheskin LJ, et al.
Evidence for exacerbation of irritable bowel syndrome during menses.
Gastroenterology. 1990 Jun. 98(6):1485-1489.

377 Singh S, Poulsom R. et al.
Cyclical constipation, is it mediated by sex steroids? Gastroenterology. 1992 April. 102(4 Part 2):A515. (Poster).

378 Crowell MD, Dubin NH, Robinson JC, et al.
Functional bowel disorders in women with dysmenorrhea.
Amer Jour Gastroenterol. 1994 Nov. 89(11):1973-7.

379 Pulkkinen MO.
Prostaglandins and the non-pregnant uterus: the pathophysiology of primary dysmenorrhea.
Acta Obstet Gynecol Scand Suppl. 1983. 113:63-7.

380 Jackson SL, Weber AM, Hull TL, et al.
Fecal incontinence in women with urinary incontinence and pelvic organ prolapse.
Obstet Gynecol. 1997 Mar. 89(3):423-7.

381 Womack NR, Morrison JFB, Williams NS.
The role of pelvic floor denervation in the aetiology of idiopathic faecal incontinence.
Brit Jour Surg. 1986 May. 73:404-7.

382 Burns DG.
The irritable bowel syndrome - a study from private practice.
S Afr Med Jour. 1985 Sept 14. 68:397-401.

383 Burns DG.
The irritable bowel syndrome - a study from private practice.
S Afr Med Jour. 1985 Sept 14. 68:397-401.

384 Prior A, Stanley KM, Smith ARB, Read NW.
Relation between hysterectomy and the irritable bowel: a prospective study.
Gut. 1992 Jun. 33(6):814-7.

385 Longstreth GF.
Irritable bowel syndrome and chronic pelvic pain.

Obstet Gynecol Survey. 1994. 49(7):505-7.

386   Gambone JC, Reiter RC.
      Nonsurgical management of chronic pelvic pain: a multidisciplinary approach.
      Clin Obstet Gynecol. 1990 Mar. 33(1):205-211.

387   Dicker RC, Greenspan JR, Strauss LT, Cowart MR, et al.
      Complications of abdominal and vaginal hysterectomy among women of reproductive age in the United States: The Collaborative Review of Sterilization.
      Amer Jour Obstet Gynecol. 1982 Dec. 144(7):841-8.
      National Center for Health Statistics: Utilization of short-stay hospitals: Annual summary for the United States.
      In: *Vital & Health Statistics.* Washington, DC. Series 13, number 128. Table 22. p 40.

388   Stovall TG, Ling FW, et al.
      Hysterectomy for chronic pelvic pain of presumed uterine etiology.
      Obstet Gynecol. 1990. 75:676-9.
      Smith RP.
      Pelvic Pain
      In: *Gynecology in Primary Care.* Baltimore, MD. Williams & Wilkins. 1997. Ch. 22. p494.

389   Burns DG.
      The irritable bowel syndrome - a study from private practice.
      S Afr Med Jour. 1985 Sept 14. 68:397-401.
      Koziol JA, Clark DC, Gittes RF, Tan EM.
      The natural history of interstitial cystitis: a survey of 374 patients.
      Jour Urology. 1993 Mar. 149:465-9.

390   Sivri A, Cindas A, Dincer F, Sivri B.
      Bowel dysfunction and irritable bowel syndrome in fibromyalgia patients.
      Clin Rheumatol. 1996. 15(3):283-6.

391   Sivri A, Cindas A, Dincer F, Sivri B.
      Bowel dysfunction and irritable bowel syndrome in fibromyalgia patients.
      Clin Rheumatol. 1996. 15(3):283-6.
      Alagiri M, Chottiner S, et al.
      Interstitial cystitis: unexplained associations with other chronic disease and pain syndromes.
      Urology. 1997. 49(suppl 5A):52-7.
      Burns DG.
      The irritable bowel syndrome - a study from private practice.
      S Afr Med Jour. 1985 Sept 14. 68:397-401.
      Koziol JA, Clark DC, Gittes RF, Tan EM.
      The natural history of interstitial cystitis: a survey of 374 patients.
      Jour Urology. 1993 Mar. 149:465-9.

Chapter 12:   Avoid Accidents

392   The Burton Goldberg Group
      Reconstructive therapy.
      In: *Alternative Medicine: The Definitive Guide.* ed. by Strohecker J, et al. Fife, WA. Future Medicine Publishing, Inc. 1995. pp434-8.

393   Fedor-Freybergh P.
      The influence of oestrogens on the wellbeing and mental performance in climacteric and postmenopausal women.

Acta Obstet Gyn Scand. 1977. 64(S):1-68.

394 Brincat M, Moniz C, Savvas M, Studd JWW.
Oestrogen deficiency and connective Tissue.
In: *HRT and Osteoporosis.* ed. by Drife JO, Studd JWW. London, England.
Springer-Verlag London Ltd. 1990. Chapter 5:47-55.

395 Holland EFN, Studd JWW, et al.
**Changes in collagen composition and cross-links in bone and skin of
osteoporotic postmenopausal women treated with percutaneous estradiol
implants.**
Obstet Gynecol. 1994 Feb. 83(2):180-3.

Smith P.
Age changes in the female urethra.
Brit Jour Urol. 1972. 44:667-676.

Brincat M, Moniz CF, et al.
Sex hormones and skin collagen content in postmenopausal women.
Brit Med Jour. 1983 Nov 5. 287:1337-8.

McConkey B, Fraser GM, et al.
Transparent skin and osteoporosis.
Lancet. 1963 Mar 30. p693-5.

Brincat M, Moniz C, Savvas M, Studd JWW.
Oestrogen deficiency and connective Tissue.
In: *HRT and Osteoporosis.* ed. by Drife JO, Studd JWW. London, England.
Springer-Verlag London Ltd. 1990. Chapter 5:47-55.

Albright F, Smith PH, Richardson AM.
Postmenopausal osteoporosis: its clinical features.
Jour Amer Med Assoc. 1941 May 31. 116(22):2465-2474.

396 Maheux R, Naud F, Rioux M, Grenier R, Lemay A, et al.
**A randomized, double-blind, placebo-controlled study on the effect of
conjugated estrogens on skin thickness.**
Amer Jour Obstet Gynecol. 1994 Feb. 170(2):642-9.

397 Minucci S, Chieffi Baccari G, Di Matteo L.
**The effect of sex hormones on lipid content and mast cell number in the
harderian gland of the female toad, Bufo viridis.**
Tissue Cell. 1994. 26(6):797-805.

398 Vander AJ, Sherman JH, Luciano DS.
Regulation of organic metabolism and energy balance.
In: *Human Physiology: The Mechanisms of Body Function.* 2nd ed. McGraw-
Hill. 1975. Ch. 13. p409.

Baird DT.
Amenorrhea, anovulation, and dysfunctional uterine bleeding.
In: *Endocrinology.* ed. by DeGroot LJ, et al. 3rd ed. Philadelphia, PA. WB
Saunders Co. 1995. Vol. 3. Ch. 118. p2072

Ehrmann DA, Barnes RB, Rosenfield.
Hyperandrogenism, hirsutism, and the polycystic ovary syndrome.
In: *Endocrinology.* ed. by DeGroot LJ, et al. 3rd ed. Philadelphia, PA. WB
Saunders Co. 1995. Vol. 3. Ch. 120. pp2093-6.

Handelsman DJ.
**Androgen physiology: testosterone and other androgens: physiology,
pharmacology and therapeutic use.**
In: *Endocrinology.* ed. by DeGroot LJ, et al. 3rd ed. Philadelphia, PA. WB
Saunders Co. 1995. Vol. 3. Ch. p2353.

399 Parker LN.
Adrenal androgens.
In: *Endocrinology.* ed. by DeGroot LJ, et al. 3rd ed. Philadelphia, PA. WB

Saunders Co. 1995. Vol. 2. Ch. 105. p1843.

400   Bhasin S, Storer TW, Berman N, Yarasheski KE, et al.
       Testosterone replacement increases fat-free mass and muscle size in
       hypogonadal men.
       Jour Clin Endocrinol Metab. 1997 Feb. 82(2):407-13.

       Wang C, Eyre DR, Clark R, Kleinberg D, Newman C, et al.
       Sublingual testosterone replacement improves muscle mass and strength,
       decreases bone resorption, and increases bone formation markers in
       hypogonadal men - A Clinical Research Center Study.
       Jour Clin Endocrinol Metab. 1996. 81(10):3654-3662.

       Urban RJ, Bodenburg YH, Gilkison C, Foxworth J, et al.
       Testosterone administration to elderly men increases skeletal muscle
       strength and protein synthesis.
       Amer Jour Physiol. 1995 Nov. 269(5 Pt 1):E820-6.

       Tenover JS.
       Effects of testosterone supplementation in the aging male.
       Jour Clin Endocrinol Metab. 1992. 75(4):1092-8.

401   Tenover JS.
       Effects of testosterone supplementation in the aging male.
       Jour Clin Endocrinol Metab. 1992. 75(4):1092-8.

402   Ishii DN, Shooter EM.
       Regulation of nerve growth factor synthesis in mouse submaxillary glands
       by testosterone.
       Jour Neurochem. 1975. 25:843-851.

       Russell WE, Van Wyk JJ.
       Peptide growth factors
       In: *Endocrinology.* ed. by DeGroot LJ, et al. 3rd ed. Philadelphia, PA. WB
       Saunders Co. 1995. Vol. 3. Ch. 142. pp2610-1.

Chapter 13:   Sexual Enjoyment

403   Masters WH, Johnson VE.
       The female orgasm.
       In: *Human sexual response.* Boston, MA. Little Brown & Co. 1966. Ch. 9.
       pp127-140.

       Masters WH, Johnson VE.
       Similarities in physiologic response.
       In: *Human sexual response.* Boston, MA. Little Brown & Co. 1966. Ch. 17.
       p288.

404   Kretzschmar NR, Gardiner S.
       A consideration of the surgical menopause after hysterectomy and the
       occurrence of cancer in the stump following subtotal hysterectomy.
       Amer Jour Obstet Gynecol. 1935. 29:168-175.

       Filiberti A, Regazzoni M, Garavoglia M, Perilli C, Alpinelli P, et al.
       Problems after hysterectomy. A comparative content analysis of 60
       interviews with cancer and non-cancer hysterectomized women.
       Eur Jour Gynaec Oncol. 1991. XII(6):445-9.

       Kilkku P, Gronroos M, Hirvonen T, Rauramo L.
       Supravaginal uterine amputation vs. hysterectomy: effects on libido and
       orgasm.

Acta Obstet Gynecol Scand. 1983. 62:147-152.

Nathorst-Boos J, von Schoultz B.

Psychological reactions and sexual life after hysterectomy with and without oophorectomy.

Gynecol Obstet Invest. 1992. 34:97-101.

Raboch J, Boudnik V, Raboch J Jr.

Sex life following hysterectomy.

Geburtshilfe Frauenheilkd. 1985 Jan. 45(1):48-50. (Abstract).

405 Nathorst-Boos J, von Schoultz B, Carlstrom K.

Elective ovarian removal and estrogen replacement therapy — effects on sexual life, psychological well-being and androgen status.

Jour Psy Obstet Gynecol. 1993 Dec. 14(4):283-93.

Chakravarti S, Collins WP, Newton JR, Oram DH, Studd JWW.

Endocrine changes and symptomatology after oophorectomy in premenopausal women.

Brit Jour Obstet Gynaecol. 1977 Oct. 84:769-775.

Lipscomb GH, Ling FW, Stovall TG, et al.

Peritoneal closure at vaginal hysterectomy: a reassessment.

Obstet Gynecol. 1996 Jan. 87(1):40-3.

Kretzschmar NR, Gardiner S.

A consideration of the surgical menopause after hysterectomy and the occurrence of cancer in the stump following subtotal hysterectomy.

Amer Jour Obstet Gynecol. 1935. 29:168-175.

Poad D, Arnold EP.**Sexual function after pelvic surgery in women.**

Aust New Zealand Jour Obstet Gynaecol. 1994. 34(4):471-4.

406 Poad D, Arnold EP.

Sexual function after pelvic surgery in women.

Aust New Zealand Jour Obstet Gynaecol. 1994. 34(4):471-4.

407 Greisheimer EM, Wiedeman MP.

Reproduction.

In: *Physiology & Anatomy.* 9th edPhiladelphia, PA. JB Lippincott Co. 1972. p612-3.

Gray H.

The urogenital system.

In: *Anatomy of the human body.* ed. by Clemente CD, Drew CR. 13th ed Philadelphia, PA. Lea & Febiger. 1985. p1518-1524.

408 Sluijmer AV, Heineman MJ, De Jong FH, Evers JLH.

Endocrine activity of the postmenopausal ovary: the effects of pituitary down-regulation and oophorectomy.

Jour Clin Endocrinol Metab. 1995 Jul. 80(7):2163-7.

Lincoln DW.

Gonadotropin-releasing hormone (GnRH): basic physiology.

In: *Endocrinology.* ed. by DeGroot LJ, et al. 3rd ed. Philadelphia, PA. WB Saunders Co. 1995. Vol 1. Ch. 13. pp218-229.

409 Sherwin BB, Gelfand MM.

The role of androgen in the maintenance of sexual functioning in oophorectomized women.

Psycho Med. 1987. 49:397-409.

Bellerose SB; Binik YM.

Body image and sexuality in oophorectomized women.

Archives of Sexual Behavior. 1993 Oct. 22(5):435-459.

Sherwin BB.

Sex hormones and psychological functioning in postmenopausal women.

Exp Gerontol. 1994. 29(3-4):423-430.

Sherwin BB, Gelfand MM, et al.

Androgen enhances sexual motivation in females: a prospective, cross over study of sex steroid administration in the surgical menopause.

Psychosom Med. 1985 Jul/Aug. 47(4):339-351.

Leiblum S, Bachmann G, Kemmann E, et al.

Vaginal atrophy in the postmenopausal woman: the importance of sexual activity and hormones.

Jour Amer Med Assoc. 1983 Apr. 249(16):2195-8.

Vander AJ, Sherman JH, Luciano DS.

Reproduction.

In: *Human Physiology: The Mechanisms of Body Function.* 2nd ed. McGraw-Hill. 1975. Ch. 14. pp436-8.

410   Sherwin BB, Gelfand MM.

The role of androgen in the maintenance of sexual functioning in oophorectomized women.

Psychosom Med. 1987. 49:397-409.

411   Nathorst-Boos J, von Schoultz B, Carlstrom K.

Elective ovarian removal and estrogen replacement therapy — effects on sexual life, psychological well-being and androgen status.

Jour Psy Obstet Gynecol. 1993 Dec. 14(4):283-93.

Bellerose SB; Binik YM.

Body image and sexuality in oophorectomized women.

Archives of Sexual Behavior. 1993 Oct. 22(5):435-459.

Nathorst-Boos J, von Schoultz B.

Psychological reactions and sexual life after hysterectomy with and without oophorectomy.

Gynecol Obstet Invest. 1992. 34:97-101.

412   Zussman L, Zussman S, Sunley R, Bjornson E.

Sexual response after hysterectomy-oophorectomy: recent studies and reconsideration of psychogenesis.

Amer Jour Obstet Gynecol. 1981 Aug 1. 140(7):725-9.

Salmon UJ, Geist SH.

Effect of androgens upon libido in women.

Jour Clin Endocrinol. 1943 Apr. 3:235-8.

413   Nathorst-Boos J, von Schoultz B.

Psychological reactions and sexual life after hysterectomy with and without oophorectomy.

Gynecol Obstet Invest. 1992. 34:97-101.

414   Nathorst-Boos J, von Schoultz B, Carlstrom K.

Elective ovarian removal and estrogen replacement therapy — effects on sexual life, psychological well-being and androgen status.

Jour Psy Obstet Gynecol. 1993 Dec. 14(4):283-93.

415   Salmon UJ, Geist SH.

Effect of androgens upon libido in women.

Jour Clin Endocrinol. 1943 Apr. 3:235-8.

Sherwin BB, Gelfand MM.

The role of androgen in the maintenance of sexual functioning in oophorectomized women.

Psychosom Med. 1987. 49:397-409.

Sherwin BB, Gelfand MM, et al.

Androgen enhances sexual motivation in females: a prospective, cross over study of sex steroid administration in the surgical menopause.

Psychosom Med. 1985 Jul/Aug. 47(4):339-351.

416   Masters WH, Johnson VE.

The female orgasm.

In: *Human sexual response.* Boston, MA. Little Brown & Co. 1966. Ch. 9. pp127-140.

Masters WH, Johnson VE.

Similarities in physiologic response.

In: *Human sexual response.* Boston, MA. Little Brown & Co. 1966. Ch. 13. p288.

Fox CA, Wolff HS, Baker JA.

Measurement of intra-vaginal and intra-uterine pressures during human coitus by radio-telemetry.

Jour Reprod Fert. 1970. 22:243-251.

417   Nathorst-Boos J, von Schoultz B.

Psychological reactions and sexual life after hysterectomy with and without oophorectomy.

Gynecol Obstet Invest. 1992. 34:97-101.

418   Zussman L, Zussman S, Sunley R, Bjornson E.

Sexual response after hysterectomy-oophorectomy: recent studies and reconsideration of psychogenesis.

Amer Jour Obstet Gynecol. 1981 Aug 1. 140(7):725-9.

419   Watson T.

Vaginal cuff closure with abdominal hysterectomy: a new approach.

Jour Reprod Med. 1994 Nov. 39(11):903-7.

420   Nathorst-Boos J, von Schoultz B.

Psychological reactions and sexual life after hysterectomy with and without oophorectomy.

Gynecol Obstet Invest. 1992. 34:97-101.

421   Zussman L, Zussman S, Sunley R, Bjornson E.

Sexual response after hysterectomy-oophorectomy: recent studies and reconsideration of psychogenesis.

Amer Jour Obstet Gynecol. 1981 Aug 1. 140(7):725-9.

422   Hendricks-Matthews MK.

The importance of assessing a woman's history of sexual abuse before hysterectomy.

The Jour Family Practice. 1991. 32(6):631-2.

423   Brahams D.

Unwanted hysterectomies.

Lancet. 1993 Aug 7. 342(8867):361.

424   Hendricks-Matthews MK.

The importance of assessing a woman's history of sexual abuse before hysterectomy.

The Jour Family Practice. 1991. 32(6):631-2.

425   Plichta SB, Abraham C.

Violence and gynecologic health in women <50 years old.

Amer Jour Obstet Gynecol. 1996 Mar. 174(3):903-7.

426   Plichta SB, Abraham C.

Violence and gynecologic health in women <50 years old.

Amer Jour Obstet Gynecol. 1996 Mar. 174(3):903-7.
Hendricks-Matthews MK.
The importance of assessing a woman's history of sexual abuse before hysterectomy.
The Jour Family Practice. 1991. 32(6):631-2.

427   Bellerose SB; Binik YM.
Body image and sexuality in oophorectomized women.
Archives of Sexual Behavior. 1993 Oct. 22(5):435-459.

428   Key FL.
Female circumcision/female genital mutilation in the United States: legislation and its implications for health providers.
JAMWA. 1997. 52(4):179-180,187.
Eyega Z, Conneely E.
Facts and fiction regarding female circumcision/female genital mutilation: a pilot study in New York city.
JAMWA. 1997. 52(4):174-8,187.

Chapter 14:   Hormone Replacement Therapy

429   Pansini F, Bonaccorsi G, et al.
Influence of spontaneous and surgical menopause on atherogenic metabolic risk.
Maturatis. 1993 Nov. 17(3):181-190.
Hreshchyshyn MM, Hopkins A, et al.
Effects of natural menopause, hysterectomy, and oophorectomy on lumbar spine and femoral neck bone densities.
Obstet Gynecol. 1988 Oct. 72(4):631-8.

430   Ernster VL, Bush TL, Huggins GR, Hulka BS, et al.
Clinical perspectives: benefits and risks of menopausal estrogen and/or progestin hormone use.
Prev. Med. 1988. 17:201-3.

431   **Cancer facts & figures - 1996.**
Atlanta, GA. American Cancer Society. 1996. Pub. 96-300M-No.5008.96:6. (Pamplet).

432   Ernster VL, Bush TL, Huggins GR, Hulka BS, et al.
Clinical perspectives: benefits and risks of menopausal estrogen and/or progestin hormone use.
Prev. Med. 1988. 17:201-3.

433   Schwartzbaum JA, Hulka BS, et al.
The influence of exogenous estrogen use on survival after diagnosis of endometrial cancer.
Amer Jour Epidemiol. 1987. 126(5):851-860.

434   Voigt LF, Weiss NS, Chu J, et al.
Progestagen supplementation of exogenous oestrogens and risk of endome-trial cancer.
Lancet. 1991 Aug 3. 338:274-7.
Persson I, Adami H, et al.
Risk of endometrial cancer after treatment with oestrogens alone or in conjunction with progestogens: results of a prospective study.

BMJ. 1989 Jan 21. 298:147-151.

435 Beral V, Bull D, Doll R, Key T, et al.
Breast cancer and hormone replacement therapy: collaborative reanalysis of data from 51 epidemiological studies of 52,705 women with breast cancer and 108,411 women without breast cancer.
Lancet. 1997 Oct 11. 350:1047-1059.

Stanford JL, Weiss NS, et al.
Combined estrogen and progestin hormone replacement therapy in relation to risk of breast cancer in middle-aged women.
Jour Amer Med Assoc. 1995. 274(2):137-142.

436 Stanford JL, Weiss NS, et al.
Combined estrogen and progestin hormone replacement therapy in relation to risk of breast cancer in middle-aged women.
Jour Amer Med Assoc. 1995. 274(2):137-142.

Dupont WD, Page DL, Rogers LW, Parl FF.
Influence of exogenous estrogens, proliferative breast disease, and other variables on breast cancer risk.
Cancer. 1989 Mar 1. 63:948-957.

437 Holli K, Isola J, Cuzick J.
Hormone replacement therapy and biological aggressiveness of breast cancer.
Lancet. 1997 Dec 6. 350:1704-5.

Beral V, Bull D, Doll R, Key T, et al.
Breast cancer and hormone replacement therapy: collaborative reanalysis of data from 51 epidemiological studies of 52,705 women with breast cancer and 108,411 women without breast cancer.
Lancet. 1997 Oct 11. 350:1047-1059.

Willis DB, Calle EE, et al.
Estrogen replacement therapy and risk of fatal breast cancer in a prospective cohort of postmenopausal women in the United States.
Cancer Causes Controls. 1996. 7:449-457.

Bergkvist L, Adami H-O, Persson I, et al.
Prognosis after breast cancer diagnosis in women exposed to estrogen and estrogen-progestogen replacement therapy.
Amer Jour Epidemiol. 1989. 130(2):221-8.

438 Steinberg KK, Thacker SB, Smith SJ, et al.
A meta-analysis of the effect of estrogen replacement therapy on the risk of breast cancer.
Jour Amer Med Assoc. 1991 Apr 17. 265(15):1985-1990.

Colditz GA, Egan KM, Stampfer MJ.
Hormone replacement therapy and risk of breast cancer: Results from epidemiologic studies.
Amer Jour Obstet Gynecol. 1993 May. 168(5):1473-1480.

Stanford JL, Weiss NS, et al.
Combined estrogen and progestin hormone replacement therapy in relation to risk of breast cancer in middle-aged women.
Jour Amer Med Assoc. 1995. 274(2):137-142.

439 Ewertz M.
Hormone therapy in the menopause and breast cancer risk - a review.

Maturitas. 1996. 23:241-6.

440   Ernster VL, Bush TL, Huggins GR, Hulka BS, et al.
        Clinical perspectives: benefits and risks of menopausal estrogen and/or
        progestin hormone use.
        Prev. Med. 1988. 17:201-3.

441   Dupont WD, Page DL, Rogers LW, Parl FF.
        Influence of exogenous estrogens, proliferative breast disease, and other
        variables on breast cancer risk.
        Cancer. 1989 Mar 1. 63:948-957.

442   Ernster VL, Bush TL, Huggins GR, Hulka BS, et al.
        Clinical perspectives: benefits and risks of menopausal estrogen and/or
        progestin hormone use.
        Prev. Med. 1988. 17:201-3.

443   Willis DB, Calle EE, et al.
        Estrogen replacement therapy and risk of fatal breast cancer in a prospec-
        tive cohort of postmenopausal women in the United States.
        Cancer Causes Controls. 1996. 7:449-457.
        Brinton LA.
        Hormone replacement therapy and risk for breast cancer.
        Endocrinol Metabol Clin North Amer. 1997 June. 26(2):361-377.

444   Willis DB, Calle EE, et al.
        Estrogen replacement therapy and risk of fatal breast cancer in a prospec-
        tive cohort of postmenopausal women in the United States.
        Cancer Causes Controls. 1996. 7:449-457.

445   Hulka BS.
        Links between hormone replacement therapy and neoplasia.
        Fertil Steril. 1994 Dec. 62(suppl 2)(6):168S-175S.

446   Chang RJ, Judd HL.
        The ovary after menopause.
        Clin Obstet Gynecol. 1981 Mar. 24(1):181-191.

447   Baird DT, Guevara A.
        Concentration of unconjugated estrone and estradiol in peripheral plasma in
        nonpregnant women throughout the menstrual cycle, castrate and postmeno-
        pausal women and in men.
        Jour Clin Endocrinol Metab. 1969 Feb. 29:149-156.

448   Baird DT, Guevara A.
        Concentration of unconjugated estrone and estradiol in peripheral plasma in
        nonpregnant women throughout the menstrual cycle, castrate and postmeno-
        pausal women and in men.
        Jour Clin Endocrinol Metab. 1969 Feb. 29:149-156.

449   Chang RJ, Judd HL.
        The ovary after menopause.
        Clin Obstet Gynecol. 1981 Mar. 24(1):181-191.
        Odell WD.
        The menopause and hormonal replacement.
        In: *Endocrinology.* ed. by DeGroot LJ, et al. 3rd ed. Philadelphia, PA. WB
        Saunders Co. 1995. Vol. 3. Ch. 122. pp2128-2139.

450   Chetkowski RJ, Meldrum DR, et al.
        Biologic effects of transdermal estradiol.
        New Engl Jour Med. 1986 June 19. 314(25):1615-1620.

451   Chetkowski RJ, Meldrum DR, et al.
        Biologic effects of transdermal estradiol.

New Engl Jour Med. 1986 June 19. 314(25):1615-1620.

Genant HK, Lucas J, Weiss S, et al.

Low-dose esterified estrogen therapy: effects on bone, plasma estradiol concentrations, endometrium, and lipid levels.

Arch Intern Med. 1997 Dec. 157:2609-2615.

Hirvonen E, Cacciatore B, Wahlstrom T, et al.

Effects of transdermal oestrogen therapy in postmenopausal women: a comparative study of an oestradiol gel and an oestradiol delivering patch.

Brit Jour Obstet Gynaecol. 1997 Nov. 104(Suppl 16):26-31.

Luisi M, Franchi F, Kicovic PM.

A group-comparative study of effects of ovestin cream versus premarin cream in post-menopausal women with vaginal atrophy.

Maturitas. 1980. 2:311-9.

Rauramo L, Punnonen R, et al.

Serum oestrone, oestradiol and oestriol concentrations in castrated women during intramuscular oestradiolvalerate and oestradiolbenzoate-ostradiolphenylpropionate therapy.

Maturitas. 1979. 2:53-8.

Nichols KC, Schenkel L, Benson H.

17β-estradiol for postmenopausal estrogen replacement therapy.

Obstet Gynecol Surv. 1984. 39(4):230-245.

452   Lyrenas S, Carlstrom K, et al.

A comparison of serum oestrogen levels after percutaneous and oral administration of oestradiol-17β.

Brit Jour Obstet Gynaecol. 1981 Feb. 88:181-7.

von Schoultz B.

Estrogens around the menopause.

Acta Obstet Gynecol Scand Suppl. 1985. 130:25-7.

453   Willis DB, Calle EE, et al.

Estrogen replacement therapy and risk of fatal breast cancer in a prospective cohort of postmenopausal women in the United States.

Cancer Causes Controls. 1996. 7:449-457.

454   von Schoultz B.

Estrogens around the menopause.

Acta Obstet Gynecol Scand Suppl. 1985. 130:25-7.

455   von Schoultz B.

Estrogens around the menopause.

Acta Obstet Gynecol Scand Suppl. 1985. 130:25-7.

456   Lyrenas S, Carlstrom K, et al.

A comparison of serum oestrogen levels after percutaneous and oral administration of oestradiol-17b.

Brit Jour Obstet Gynaecol. 1981 Feb. 88:181-7.

457   von Schoultz B.

Estrogens around the menopause.

Acta Obstet Gynecol Scand Suppl. 1985. 130:25-7.

Varma TR, Everard D, Hole D.

Effect of natural estrogen on the serum level of follicle-stimulating hormone (FSH), estradiol and estrone in post-menopausal women and its effect on endometrium.

Acta Obstet Gynecol Scand. 1985. 64:105-9.

Mattsson L, Cullberg G, Samsioe G.

Influence of esterified estrogens and medroxyprogesterone on lipid metabolism and sex steroids: a study in oophorectomized women.

Horm Metabol Res. 1982 Nov. 14(11):602-6.

458   Carr BR, MacDonald PC.
      The menopause and beyond.
      In: *Principles of Geriatric Medicine.* ed by Andres R, et al. New York. McGraw-
      Hill Book Company. 1985. Ch. 31. p333.
      von Schoultz B.
      Estrogens around the menopause.
      Acta Obstet Gynecol Scand Suppl. 1985. 130:25-7.

459   Edmondson HA, Reynolds TB, Henderson B, Benton B.
      Regression of liver cell adenomas associated with oral contraceptives.
      Ann Intern Med. 1977 Feb. 86(2):180-2.

460   **Premarin®: vaginal cream.**
      In: *Physicians' Desk Reference.* 52nd Ed. Medical Economics Company, Inc.
      Montvale, NJ. 1998. p3115.

461   **Premarin®: vaginal cream.**
      In: *Physicians' Desk Reference.* 52nd Ed. Medical Economics Company, Inc.
      Montvale, NJ. 1998. p3115.

462   von Schoultz B.
      Estrogens around the menopause.
      Acta Obstet Gynecol Scand Suppl. 1985. 130:25-7.
      Premarin®
      In: *Physicians' Desk Reference.* 52nd Ed. Medical Economics Company, Inc.
      Montvale, NJ. 1998. pp3111-5.
      Godsland IF, Gangar K, Walton C, et al.
      **Insulin resistance, secretion, and elimination in postmenopausal women
      receiving oral or transdermal hormone replacement therapy.**
      Metabolism. 1993 Jul. 42(7):846-853.
      Slemenda C, Longcope C, Peacock M, Hui S, Johnston CC.
      **Sex steroids, bone mass, and bone loss: A prospective study of pre-, peri-,
      and postmenopausal women.**
      Journ Clin Invest. 1996 Jan 1. 97(1):14-21.
      Chetkowski RJ, Meldrum DR, et al.
      Biologic effects of transdermal estradiol.
      New Engl Jour Med. 1986 June 19. 314(25):1615-1620.
      The Writing group for the PEPI trial.
      **Effects of estrogen or estrogen/progestin regimens on heart disease risk
      factors in postmenopausal women: the postmenopausal estrogen/progestin
      interventions (PEPI) trail.**
      Jour Amer Med Assoc. 1995 Jan 18. 273(3):199-208.

463   Holst J, Cajander S, et al.
      **A comparison of liver protein induction in postmenopausal women during
      oral and percutaneous oestrogen replacement therapy.**
      Brit Jour Obstet Gynaecol. 1983 Apr. 90:355-360.
      O'Connell MB.
      **Pharmacokinetic and pharmacologic variation between different estrogen
      products.**
      Jour Clin Pharmacol. 1995 Sept. 35(suppl):18S-24S.

464   Greenblatt RB, Natrajan PK, et al.
      **The fate of a large bolus of exogenous estrogen administered to postmeno-
      pausal women.**
      Maturitas. 1979. 2:29-35.
      Sitruk-Ware R, de Lignieres B, Basdevant A, Mauvais-Jarvis P.
      Absorption of percutaneous oestradiol in postmenopausal women.

Maturitas. 1980. 2:207-211.

465 Habiba M, Andrea A, et al.
Thrombophilia and lipid profile in post-menopausal women using a new transdermal oestradiol patch.
Eur Jour Obstet Gynecol Repro Biol. 1996. 66:165-8.

Palacios S, Menendez C, et al.
Effects of oestradiol administration via different routes on the lipid profile in women with bilateral oophorectomy.
Maturitas. 1994. 18:239-244.

Castelo-Branco C, Casals E, et al.
Effects of oophorectomy and hormone replacement therapy on plasma lipids.
Maturitas. 1993. 17:113-122.

466 Palacios S, Menendez C, et al.
Effects of oestradiol administration via different routes on the lipid profile in women with bilateral oophorectomy.
Maturitas. 1994. 18:239-244.

Everson SA, Matthews KA, et al.
Effects of surgical menopause on psychological characteristics and lipid levels: the healthy women study.
Health Psychol. 1995. 14(5):435-443.

Castelo-Branco C, Casals E, et al.
Effects of oophorectomy and hormone replacement therapy on plasma lipids.
Maturitas. 1993. 17:113-122.

467 Clarkson TB.
Estrogens, progestins, and coronary heart disease in cynomolgus monkeys.
Fertil Steril. 1994 Dec. 62(Suppl 2)6:147S-151S.

468 Godsland IF, Gangar K, Walton C, et al.
Insulin resistance, secretion, and elimination in postmenopausal women receiving oral or transdermal hormone replacement therapy.
Metabolism. 1993 Jul. 42(7):846-853.

469 Reaven GM.
Role of insulin resistance in human disease.
Diabetes. 1988 Dec. 37:1595-1607.

Winocour PH, Kaluvya S, Ramaiya K, et al.
Relation between insulinemia, body mass index, and lipoprotein composition in healthy, nondiabetic men and women.
ArteriosclerThromb. 1992 Mar. 12(3):393-402.

Peiris AN, Sothmann MS, et al.
Adiposity, fat distribution, and cardiovascular risk.
Annals Internal Med. 1989 Jun 1. 110(11):867-872.

Shinozaki K, Hattori Y, Suzuki M, et al.
Insulin resistance as an independent risk factor for carotid artery wall intima media thickening in vasospastic angina.
Arterioscl Thromb Vasc Biol. 1997 Nov. 17(11):3302-3310.

470 Lufkin EG, Wahner HW, O'Fallon WM, Hodgson SF, et al.
Treatment of postmenopausal osteoporosis with transdermal estrogen.
Ann Intern Med. 1992 July 1. 117(1):1-9.

Lufkin EG, Riggs BL.
Three-year follow-up on effects of transdermal estrogen.

Ann Intern Med. 1996 July 1. 125(1):77.

471   Dickerson J, Bressler R, Christian CD, Hermann HW.
Efficacy of estradiol vaginal cream in postmenopausal women.
Clin Pharmacol Ther. 1979 Oct. 26(4):502-7.

472   **TestodermC III (testosterone transdermal system)**
Palo Alto, CA. Alza Pharmaceuticals. 6/94 Ed. (Package insert).

473   **TestodermC III (testosterone transdermal system)**
Palo Alto, CA. Alza Pharmaceuticals. 6/94 Ed. (Package insert).

474   Bellerose SB; Binik YM.
Body image and sexuality in oophorectomized women.
Archives of Sexual Behavior. 1993 Oct. 22(5):435-459.

475   Potischman N, Falk RT, et al.
Reproducibility of laboratory assays for steroid hormones and sex hormone-binding globulin.
Cancer Res. 1994 Oct 15. 54:5363-7.

Hankinson SE, Manson JE, et al.
Laboratory reproducibility of endogenous hormone levels in postmeno-pausal women.
Cancer Epidemiol Bio Prev. 1994 Jan/Feb. 3:51-6.

476   Rees MCP.
The need to improve compliance to HRT.
Brit Jour Obstet Gynaecol. 1997 Nov. 104(suppl 16):1-3.

Sulak PJ.
Endometrial cancer and hormone replacement therapy.
Endocrinol Metabol Clin North Amer. 1997 June. 26(2):399-411.

Chapter 15: Social, Medical, Political and Economic Institutions

477   Weiner MF, Vobach S, Olsson K, Svetlik D, Risser RC.
Cortisol secretion and Alzheimer's disease progression.
Biol Psychiatry. 1997. 42:1030-8.

478   Fillit H, Weinreb H, et al.
Observations in a preliminary open trial of estradiol therapy for senile dementia-Alzheimer's type.
Psychoneuroendocrinology. 1986. 11(3):337-345.

479   Simpkins JW, Green PS, Gridley KE, Singh M, et al.
Role of estrogen replacement therapy in memory enhancement and the prevention of neuronal loss associated with Alzheimer's disease.
Amer Jour Med. 1997 Sept 22. 103(3A):19S-25S.

Tang M, Jacobs D, et al.
Effect of oestrogen during menopause on risk and age at onset of Alzheimer's disease.
Lancet. 1996 Aug 17. 348:429-432.

Paganini-Hill A, Henderson VW.
Estrogen replacement therapy and risk of Alzheimer disease.
Arch Intern Med. 1996 Oct 28. 156:2213-7.

Resnick SM, Metter EJ, Zonderman AB.
Estrogen replacement therapy and longitudinal decline in visual memory: a possible protective effect?
Neurology. 1997. 49:1491-7.

Henderson VW, Watt L, Buckwalter JG.
Cognitive skills associated with estrogen replacement in women with Alzheimer's disease.

Psychoneuroendocrinology. 1996. 21(4):421-430.

480   Tagawa H, Shimokawa H, Tagawa T, et al.
Short-term estrogen augments both nitric oxide-mediated and non-nitric oxide-mediated endothelium-dependent forearm vasodilation in postmenopausal women.
Jour Cardiovasc Pharmacol. 1997. 30(4):481-8.

Toran-Allerand CD, Miranda RC, et al.
Estrogen receptors colocalize with low-affinity nerve growth factor receptors in cholinergic neurons of the basal forebrain.
Proc Natl Acad Sci USA. 1992 May. 89:4668-4672.

Fillit H.
Future therapeutic developments of estrogen use.
Jour Clin Pharmacol. 1995 Sept. 35(Sept Suppl):25S-28S.

Simpkins JW, Green PS, Gridley KE, Singh M, et al.
Role of estrogen replacement therapy in memory enhancement and the prevention of neuronal loss associated with Alzheimer's disease.
Amer Jour Med. 1997 Sept 22. 103(3A):19S-25S.

481   **Alzheimer's disease statistics fact sheet.**
Alzheimer's Association, Inc. 1995. Modified: 1996 Nov. 19. (Internet).

482   Hagstad A, Janson PO.
The epidemiology of climacteric symptoms.
Acta Obstet Gynecol Scand Suppl. 1986. 134:59-65.

Barlow DH, Brockie JA, Rees CMP.
Study of general practice consultations and menopausal problems.
BMJ. 1991 Feb 2. 302:274-6.

Thompson B, Hart SA, Durno D.
Menopausal age and symptomatology in general practice.
Jour Biosoc Sci. 1973. 5:71-82.

Lock M, Kaufert P, Gilbert P.
Cultural construction of the menopausal syndrome: the Japanese case.
Maturitas. 1988. 10:317-332.

Boulet MJ, Oddens BJ, et al.
Climacteric and menopause in seven south-east Asian countries.
Maturitas. 1994. 19:157-176.

Haines CJ, Rong L, et al.
The perception of the menopause and the climacteric among women in Hong Kong and southern China.
Prevent Med. 1995. 24:245-8.

483   Haines CJ, Chung TKH, Leung DHY.
A prospective study of the frequency of acute menopausal symptoms in Hong Kong Chinese women.
Maturitas. 1994. 18:175-181.

484   Kao PC, P'eng FK.
How to reduce the risk factors of osteoporosis in Asia.
Chung-Hua i Hsueh Tsa Chih Chinese Med Jour. (Taipei) 1995 Mar. 55(3):209-212.

Knight DC, Eden JA.
Phytoestrogens - a short review.
Maturitas. 1995. 22:167-175.

485   Kao PC, P'eng FK.
How to reduce the risk factors of osteoporosis in Asia.
Chung-Hua i Hsueh Tsa Chih Chinese Med Jour. (Taipei) 1995 Mar. 55(3):209-

        212.
486   **Cancer rates and risks.**
        US Dept of Health and Human Services, Public Health Service, National
        Institutes of Health. 1996. (Pamphlet).
487   Yip CH, Ng EH.
        **Breast cancer - a comparative study between Malaysian and Singaporean
        women.**
        Singapore Med Jour. 1996. 37:264-267.
        Seow A, Duffy SW, McGee MA, Lee J, Lee HP.
        Breast cancer in Singapore: trends in incidence 1968-1992.
        Int Jour Epidemiol. 1996. 25(1):40-45.
488   Lee HP, Day NE, Shanmugaratnam K.
        Trends in cancer incidence in Singapore 1968-1982.
        Singapore Cancer Registry. WHO. IARC Scientific Pub. No. 91. 1988.
489   Ng E, Gao F, Ji C, Ho G, Soo K.
        **Risk factors for breast carcinoma in Singaporean Chinese women: the role
        of central obesity.**
        Cancer. 1997 Aug 15. 80(4):725-731.
490   Ng E, Gao F, Ji C, Ho G, Soo K.
        **Risk factors for breast carcinoma in Singaporean Chinese women: the role
        of central obesity.**
        Cancer. 1997 Aug 15. 80(4):725-731.
491   Knight DC, Eden JA.
        Phytoestrogens - a short review.
        Maturitas. 1995. 22:167-175.
492   **Cancer facts & figures - 1996.**
        Atlanta, GA. American Cancer Society. 1996. Pub. 96-300M-No.5008.96:6.
        (Pamplet).
493   Miller NF.
        Hysterectomy: therapeutic necessity or surgical racket?
        Amer Jour Obstet Gynecol. 1946. 51: 804-810.
494   **National Center for Health Statistics: Utilization of short-stay hospitals:
        Annual summary for the United States.**
        In: *Vital & Health Statistics.* Washington, DC. Series 13, number 31. Table 23. p
        54.
495   Gambone JC, Reiter RC, Lench JF, Moore JG.
        **The impact of a quality assurance process on the frequency and confirma-
        tion rate of hysterectomy.**
        Amer Jour Obstet Gynecol. 1990 Aug. 163:545-550.
496   Mc Carthy EG, Finkel ML.
        Second consultant opinion for elective gynecologic surgery.
        Obstet Gynecol. 1980 Oct. 56(4):403-410.
497   Bernstein SJ, McGlynn EA, Siu AL, et al.
        **The appropriateness of hysterectomy: a comparison of care in seven health
        plans.**
        Jour Amer Med Assoc. 1993 May 12. 269(18):2398-2402.
498   Wood C, Maher P, Hill D, Selwood T.
        Hysterectomy: a time of change.
        Med Jour Aust. 1992 Nov 16. 157:651-3.
        Browne DS, Frazer MI.
        Hysterectomy Revisited.

Aust New Zealand Jour Obstet Gynaecol. 1991. 31(2)148-152.

Dicker RC, Greenspan JR, Strauss LT, Cowart MR, et al.

Complications of abdominal and vaginal hysterectomy among women of reproductive age in the United States: The Collaborative Review of Sterilization.

Amer Jour Obstet Gynecol. 1982 Dec. 144(7):841-8.

Weber AM, Lee J.

Use of alternative techniques of hysterectomy in Ohio, 1988-1994.

New Engl Jour Med. 1996 Aug 15. 335(7):483-9.

Meikle SF, Ungent EW, Orleans M.

Complications and recovery from laparoscopy-assisted vaginal hysterectomy compared with abdominal and vaginal hysterectomy.

Obstet Gynecol. 1997 Feb. 89(2):304-311.

Boike GM, Elfstrand EP, DelPriore G, Schumock D, et al.

Laparoscopically assisted vaginal hysterectomy in a university hospital: report of 82 cases and comparison with abdominal and vaginal hysterectomy.

Amer Jour Obstet Gynecol. 1993. 168(6)(Part 1):1690-1701.

Nezhat C, Bess O, Admon D, Nezhat CH, Nezhat F.

Hospital cost comparison between abdominal, vaginal, and laparoscopy-assisted vaginal hysterectomies.

Obstet Gynecol. 1994 May. 83(5 part 1):713-6.

Dorsey JH, Holtz PM, Griffiths RI, McGrath MM, Steinberg EP.

Costs and charges associated with three alternative techniques of hysterectomy.

New Engl Jour Med. 1996 Aug 15. 335(7):476-482.

Harris MB, Olive DL.

Changing hysterectomy patterns after introduction of laparoscopically assisted vaginal hysterectomy.

Amer Jour Obstet Gynecol. 1994 Aug. 171(2):340-4.

499   Harris MB, Olive DL.

Changing hysterectomy patterns after introduction of laparoscopically assisted vaginal hysterectomy.

Amer Jour Obstet Gynecol. 1994 Aug. 171(2):340-4.

Weber AM, Lee J.

Use of alternative techniques of hysterectomy in Ohio, 1988-1994.

New Engl Jour Med. 1996 Aug 15. 335(7):483-9.

500   Harris MB, Olive DL.

Changing hysterectomy patterns after introduction of laparoscopically assisted vaginal hysterectomy.

Amer Jour Obstet Gynecol. 1994 Aug. 171(2):340-4.

Weber AM, Lee J.

Use of alternative techniques of hysterectomy in Ohio, 1988-1994.

New Engl Jour Med. 1996 Aug 15. 335(7):483-9.

501   Harris MB, Olive DL.

Changing hysterectomy patterns after introduction of laparoscopically assisted vaginal hysterectomy.

Amer Jour Obstet Gynecol. 1994 Aug. 171(2):340-4.

Chapter 16:   Whole Body = Whole Functioning

502   Vander AJ, Sherman JH, Luciano DS.
       Hormone control mechanisms.
       In: *Human Physiology: The Mechanisms of Body Function.* 2nd ed. McGraw-
       Hill. 1975. Ch. 7. p173.
503   Amirikia H, Evans TN.
       Ten-year review of hysterectomies: trends, indications, and risks.
       Amer Jour Obstet Gynecol. 1979 Jun. 134(4):431-7.
504   Newton N, Baron E.
       Reactions to hysterectomy: Fact or fiction?
       Primary Care. 1976 Dec. 3(4):781-801.
505   **National Center for Health Statistics: Utilization of short-stay hospitals:**
       Annual summary for the United States.
       In: *Vital & Health Statistics.* Washington, DC. Series 13, number 128. Table 22.
       p 40.

Index